Love, Hope, Faith

Love, Hope, Faith

◆

A Personal Journey Through Cancer

Gaynel Gunderson

iUniverse, Inc.
New York Lincoln Shanghai

Love, Hope, Faith
A Personal Journey Through Cancer

iUniverse books may be ordered through booksellers or by contacting:

iUniverse
2021 Pine Lake Road, Suite 100
Lincoln, NE 68512
www.iuniverse.com
1-800-Authors (1-800-288-4677)

ISBN: 0-595-34374-0

Printed in the United States of America

In Remembrance of:

Neil Rogers, my brother, whose story is told within this book.

And to my husband's sister, Audrey Gunderson-Hurst. She lost her battle with breast cancer, but she gained total healing in Christ by accepting His gift of eternal life.

Oh, what perfect, healthy, heavenly bodies you both have now!

Contents

Acknowledgments

Mary Rogers. We walked this road together with our fears and tears, only imagining the worse, then to have it happen. We loved him and lost him, but he gained all. Only his body died; he still lives. He just moved, and some day we'll move there too. What you put on the headstone is so true; "Those who live in God, never see each other for the last time." I love that.

Rory Lewellyn. To me, a servant and teacher of the Lord. Thank you for your prayers during this journey, and for making sure I was not off the mark.

Mount Si High School and Joe Dockery, teacher of *Digital Imaging Production,* and students Jessica Blessard and Bryce Saffell; my husband, Jed, said I needed a book cover showing that we can rise above the dark cloud of cancer and you truly did captured that in your book cover design.

Bob Smith. Thank you. Every man needs a good Christian friend; I'm glad you are Keith's.

Especially to my family. I was so consumed with Neil's cancer that I wasn't always there for you, and you were hurting too. You let me do what I needed to do, and you gave me the strength to do it, by loving me and supporting me. Through it all, we've cried, prayed, endured and grown. Jed, Lia, Jason, Gary and families, you are awesome!

God Bless you, one and all.

Romans 12:12…rejoicing in hope, persevering in tribulation, devoted to prayer,

Prologue

I have three older brothers, but I was raised with only one of them. My two oldest brothers were thirteen and fifteen when I was born, so by the time I was five, they were off to college. I never really got to know them until I was grown myself.

Neil was five years older than me and was the brother I grew up with.
I suppose our relationship was typical enough. I was the little sister always in the way and trying to tag along with him and his friends. He'd call me a pest and tell me to get lost and I'd stick my tongue out at him. Yet he was always there when I needed him and he'd always take care of me when the need arose. As we grew older we became 'friends', sharing feelings and confidences.

When Neil was in high school he joined the Naval Reserves and when he finished school he continued serving his country while stationed in Hawaii. This was during the Viet Nam War and I had a friend that lost her brother in that war, so I was very happy that Neil was safe in Hawaii. I often wondered how our lives might have been changed for the worse had he been sent to Viet Nam. I was so happy when he safely returned.

It didn't take long after that when he met and fell in love with Mary. He not only fell in love with her, but also her three children. Most men would be overwhelmed at taking on three children, but Neil loved those kids so much, and was so family minded that he didn't hesitate to adopt them and make them a part of our family. When Neil and Mary's son was born, this didn't take away from his love for his other three kids; it just added to it and made his family a complete circle.

After we each married and had our own families, we were still close, but we had our own roads to travel with our families and different sets of friends. Although we didn't socialize too much together, we did remain close since we worked together and saw each other five days a week. Most of the time this was great, but sometimes trying, as families can be. I'm sure there were times when we were ticked off and did not 'like' each other very much, but the deep love we grew up with was always there. He was my big brother and I was his little sister. That says it all.

Longevity was something I suppose we expected in our family. There were four of us kids who married and added twelve grandchildren and twenty-nine great grandchildren. With all of these, good health prevailed. But, as we traveled down our road of life, we've faced death in several forms.

A couple of us have lost unborn grandchildren in miscarriage. A child lost; a member of our family that we have not been privileged to get to know, but still we grieve for. Our most devastating moment came on October 17, 1985 when a drunk driver took the life of our eighteen-year-old nephew, Mark. In the flash of a moment, he was gone. We were all left with the shock of it for years to come. Our parents lived into their eighties, and although it was so very difficult to lose them, it was also a natural event because they had lived long and full lives.

We have faced death in these three ways, an unknown yet loved baby, an instant death that stole a loved one from us without prior warning, and the expected death of the aged. We had never, in our most immediate family, faced a killing disease. We were just too healthy and truly blessed in many ways to ever expect such a cross to bear.

And so, at the age of 50, I began this journey with my beloved brother Neil and his wife Mary.

1

Eulogy

Let me begin with the end by letting you read the eulogy that was written and told by our family friend.

~Neil Rogers~

As I was looking around this familiar old sanctuary earlier, I saw many friends of Neil that I know have wonderful stories to tell about him. In those stories are statements that have affected and changed many of our lives for the better. Neil Rogers got along with all sorts of people from all different walks of life. Neil was always interested in people, and when you met him you just liked him straight away and later it usually turned into a great friendship. Neil was a successful businessman but never did he put on any airs and graces that sometimes business leaders have. Neil had time for everyone and anyone and that clearly shows up today as you look at the people here who have come to pay homage to this man of gentle persuasion.

Neil and I have been together on four fronts. One, he is my good friend. Two, I worked for Neil and he was my boss. Three, because our families have dual ownership of some commercial property, we are business partners. Four, and the most important, we are brothers in Christ.

My first remembrances of Neil were at this very church. And it was never Neil alone; it was always—as it should be—Neil and Mary. They were each others' soul mate and anyone who met them instantly knew that was the way it was. You got Neil, you got Mary and vice versa and they are a perfect fit. So when I talk today about Neil remember you cannot talk about Neil in the singular because Mary was so much a part of his life they were almost inseparable.

Neil Rogers was a husband, father, grandfather, brother, brother-in-law, uncle, friend and employer. He carried out all these functions in a quiet, loving, caring and Christian manner. His marriage and family life were certainly Christian based and it showed clearly in his relationship with all of his family members. Neil was a father who always made time for his kids. As a grandfather he always made time to give his children a respite and take on his grandchildren whenever the need arose. This is how he supported his children while they taught their children to know the Lord.

Neil loved prayer. Never could you start a meeting at work, at home, or a trip without first saying and being in prayer. It was easy for Neil's employees to love and respect him. Neil allowed his employees to grow in their job. He had a faith that the right employee had been provided to him and it was Neil's job to let the employee apply their creativity to whatever position they were hired for.

All of my family came to know Neil through our various church groups and functions here at Our Lady of Sorrows and we became closer friends when we both joined the Cursillo movement, which is a Christian movement set up through the Catholic Church. The Cursillo movement is made up of small groups of men and women meeting weekly in local restaurants. We would all meet on Friday morning real early at the Mar-T café in North Bend. The first question to Neil, as it was to all of us; how did your week go? And Neil would always say, "I had a great week." I will always remember his positive answers to your questions of him. That was also his way of putting you at ease and making you feel good yourself.

I remember Neil clearly telling me, "You know what I really like? I love to just sit in a group and listen to people talk about how they came to Christ." That was Neil. He was also a great people watcher as well. I remember a few times we would go with our wives to Nordstrom to shop. Neil and I would let the girls go off to empty our wallets, and we would sit together on a seat and listen to the piano player and just watch people coming and going. We did not have to say any thing, we would just sit and watch. These simple things in life were relaxing to Neil, no need for chatter, he was just being comfortable in himself.

Neil, along with Mary, took on the teaching of some of Our Lady of Sorrows grade school children and taught them how the love of the Lord in their life could make a difference. Neil always enjoyed talking about the kids, their innocence, and his love of teaching those youngsters. Neil had a gentle way that kids responded to and I just know those kids and their parents will always remember Neil. Just look at Neil's grandchildren today and you will see the good seeds this man has sown.

As I said earlier, Neil was my boss. When I was hired to work at Truck Town, I worked for him there for about fourteen months and then was offered the chance to open Truck Town's new truck stop in Prosser. For me this was a big step. Neil had faith that I would do the job and that faith he had in me and others made us all perform well.

Neil was an extremely generous man and shared everything he had in many ways. He liked to share behind the scenes; he did not want the fanfare of people knowing when and how he was helping others out. When my relatives and friends from England came to visit, they were always invited by Neil to spend time at the beach. Neil and Mary not only lent us the beach house but they also became a part of those friendships. When Neil Rogers was your friend, it was automatic that your friends also became Neil and Mary's friends. That is the way it was, and is. Mary and Neil would even sleep on the couch in the living room at the beach and give up their own bedroom for a person they had just met.

Neil always found time for everyone in his life. That is why during the last month of Neil's life his family bedroom was the gathering place for so many people. Neil was so loved that his bedroom was like Grand Central Station. Seeing Neil there in bed was hard for all of us, and I believe he knew that. Never once in this last eleven months did I hear Neil say or complain, "Why me?" Neil loved all of us too much to complain to us, and it just wasn't his style.

Today is just another example of Neil's appeal. Neil has many friends from many walks of life. Recently I sent an email to all the member truck stops, in our Ambest truck stop group, to let them know that Neil was very sick. I received a reply from many members but I remember one in particular from a very influential man on the national scene for the truck stop industry. In his email he mentioned that Neil Rogers was a true gentleman. That is exactly how his contemporary truck stop owners refer to Neil. Neil was the past president of the Western Association of Truck Stop Operators, whose membership consists of truck stop owners on the West Coast from here in Washington and all the way down to Nevada.

Neil along with his brother Hadley, also won the State of Washington Small Business Award. No small feat for any businessman.

Many years ago when I first came to this country and settled in North Bend, I remember asking my wife Ellen, who was a bank employee in North Bend, "Where do you go for lunch?" She said, "Truck Town." I said, "You mean to tell me you go and sit down with a bunch of truckers to have lunch?" Ellen informed me that at Truck Town there was a new Ken's Restaurant, which catered to the trucker, the tourist and the locals. The food was great and it was served very quickly. Neil's touch was in that early restaurant and in the managers and all the employees. It was the same touch that every one of us has experienced with Neil, whether we were at his home in North Bend, his beach house, at a restaurant with him or at a weekend Cursillo retreat where he worked the kitchen crew. His hospitality was enormous and unforgettable.

I remember very well the first Cursillo three-day retreat where new Cursillo candidates would join our membership. Neil and I were selected for the Palanca group there, and we would take shifts praying that the three-day retreat would be a great success that would bring all the new candidates closer to Christ. When Neil and I arrived, we found out that two cooks had not shown up and the Head Cook was really upset and annoyed because all his planning was now up in the air. He was now looking at doing all the cooking, the dishes and laying out of the dining room all by himself for about eighty people. Someone suggested that the Palanca team should supply a couple of guys for the kitchen. Neil and I volunteered and we were now on kitchen crew. We did not meet the Head Cook that night, as he was asleep. They just told us to make sure we got up at 5:00 a.m. and go to the kitchen. At five a.m. off we go to the kitchen and the Head Cook is there and he isn't talking. He's still miffed about losing two experienced cooks and getting a couple of prayer partners who probably only had experience cooking in their kitchen at home. Neil took a look around and started to work. Neil told me to start making coffee and off we go. I took an interest in watching the Head Cook while I was making the coffee. He was a portly guy whom Neil and I later christened "Chef Boy R Dee." He still was not saying anything but was closely watching Neil over the grill and suddenly he realized the Lord had sent him not only a cook, but also an organized prayerful cook and maybe the weekend retreat in the kitchen had been saved after all. I watched Neil and Chef Boy R Dee interact that whole weekend and Neil changed the attitude of that man of little faith into a wonderful sharing man. We had a great time in that kitchen and

Neil applied his personal touch to decorating the dining room and cooking those meals. Those candidates had something to talk about when they got home to their wives. Every Cursillo retreat after that, Chef Boy R Dee was always there looking and asking, "where's Neil?" And they would always have the greatest time together. This was a classic Neil Rogers story, the quiet gentle person of much persuasion.

It would be remiss of me to forget Neil's wonderful sense of humor. I remember one of our many visits to the beach together and we were playing pinochle. Most of you know when you went to the beach, it was always the guys versus the gals. I am not the greatest of card players and was never one to push up the bid and take a chance unless I had all the aces and a double pinochle in my hand. I passed as usual and the girls won the bid. I laid down my meld and just looking at my meld Neil said, "Why didn't you go?" I just didn't feel I had enough. He then leans over the table looks me right in the eye and said, "And I have you running my truck stop in Prosser?"

I don't remember Neil ever putting himself first. His family was always first and Neil did whatever he could to protect them now and for the future. Two days before Valentine's Day he could not get up out of bed by himself due to his swollen stomach. He could not talk on the phone properly because of the fluid in his lungs. Again, not thinking of his own problems, he had Kenny make sure that he ordered a bouquet of flowers for Mary on Valentine's Day. To Neil it was natural to think of others above himself and in that he was a teacher to us all.

For Mary and all the Rogers family, I know there is nothing I can say that can take away your pain. Nobody knows more than Neil does, the hurts you are feeling right now. But as Neil smiles down on us today, please accept the truth that he is in heaven and is about to have his feet washed by our Lord and Savior Jesus Christ.

As I was typing this up and coming to the end of my statements, I just had this super strong feeling that I know Neil would have wanted me to say on his behalf to his immediate care givers over the last eleven months, "Thank you to the gallant doctors and nurses of Virginia Mason, the hospice nurses, my loving wife Mary, my sister Gaynel and my brother-in-law Jed for being there with me through all of the medical ups and downs of the last eleven months. And to the many prayer warriors led by my brother Hadley that sacrificed for me. I want you all to know it was not in vain.

Finally, Neil's legacy to all of us was in his actions in life. Be loving husbands, be good fathers, grandfathers, brothers and above all else, "Love God." Remember, as Neil did, the Cursillo motto as you play out your life; Make a friend, Be a friend, Bring a friend to Christ.

I have never been concerned about Neil's salvation. To me that has always been a given. Today I say goodbye to my friend and say, "Neil, be assured that everyone here will do their very best to lessen the load on Mary and your loving family as we absolutely know you would have done for each of us if the roles had been reversed."

Sincerely written by Les Cole, in Christ Jesus' Name.

2

The Phone Call and God's Guiding Hand

Neil called me on my 50th birthday. Although there had been a party for me the weekend before, I thought he just wanted to say happy birthday. It was one of those phone calls that leave you with a sense of the unknown and dread. He said he'd been having some tests and wanted me to know that they found a spot on his liver and he was going in to have further testing done. He and Mary were going to Virginia Mason Clinic in Seattle on Friday. I immediately asked him if I could go with them. For Neil to have called me with this news I knew he was very concerned and I knew I had to be there with them. And so, at this first appointment in Seattle, we became each other's support team.

I live about 150 miles from them and drove over the night before and stayed with my daughter. That morning when I arrived at Neil and Mary's we joined hands and prayed before we began 'our day'. As the day progressed, God wove us through a number of obstacles. Our appointment was with the wrong doctor for what we needed done, and without an appointment that would take weeks, we were pretty much planning to go home. Somehow, God opened the doors. Because of the compassion of the wrong doctor, who contacted the correct doctor, who squeezed Neil in, we were able to keep a nonexistent appointment. The power of prayer! It was a long anxious day that ended in Dr. B's office with him explaining to us that Neil had a cancerous tumor on his liver that probably originated in his pancreas. We were to come back on Monday for a procedure where Dr. B would actually scope inside to see what was going on.

Dr. B later referred to this day as black Friday, but Monday was the black day for us, because when we left there on Friday, we had no inkling of what we were facing. I don't think any of us even knew what the pancreas was, let alone what pancreatic cancer could mean. It was a quiet ride home with the attitude of we'll wait and see what they find on Monday. I drove back home to be with my husband for the weekend knowing I would be back Sunday night for the appointment on Monday.

I couldn't let it sit until Monday, so I got on the internet and looked up pancreatic cancer and my world fell apart. My world stopped.

3

The Fatal News; God's Promises and Strength

At some point in this March of 2000 I began to write a personal journal. I will use that journal now (written in italics) to tell this story, and fill in as needed to elaborate.

March 2000. I've had this journal now for 15 months. I've often thought to write in it. I've even taken it on trips with me but haven't written a word. Now, I'll use it to record my journey with the battle we face in Neil's cancer. I say that "we" face it, because if Neil has cancer then we all have it. (I do not mean this literally) For we are a family and what happens to one happens to all, whether sad or glad.

Neil said he was easily tired and attributed that to stress at work, and he felt ill with stomach pains when he ate.

Neil wanted to make sure nothing was wrong, because he and Mary were going on an anxiously awaited cruise. They were flying to Chili and then cruising through the Panama Canal. He was really looking forward to it and wanted to make sure he wasn't going to be sick on the trip. So he scheduled his first of several doctors' appointments, which lead us to that appointment in Seattle on Friday.

Tests showed a tumor on his liver. After his appointment on Friday I went home for the weekend. At home on Saturday I looked up pancreatic cancer on the internet. I was devastated! The secular and medical world left no hope. Everyone died of it. How do I possibly describe that feeling of total loss and helplessness? I say helpless not hopeless. There is always hope with God.

Saturday and Sunday were days of devastation and tears. I remember telling my husband what I had found, and him holding me, while we both cried. As I look back now, I know that was when the mourning process had begun. And I began to pray, really pray.

We were raised Christian, but none of us made a full commitment to the Lord until we were adults. I prayed every day for my family and friends, but when this happened to Neil everything changed. I prayed constantly and all my prayers revolved around him, and everything related to him and this battle. I went to church that Sunday morning and as soon as we started to sing the first song, I started crying and knew I wouldn't stop. I left immediately and went home, crying all the way and for most of the day. Every time I went to church after that the same thing would happen; sometimes I would start crying before I even got there. It was several months before I could stay. If I made it through the music, I was doing well, because I have always been touched by the Lord through music and I know now that this was when He started to minister to me and prepare me for what was to come.

Monday. I went with Neil and Mary to Virginia Mason. Dr. B was going to do a procedure with a scope down Neil's throat through his stomach and into the pancreas, check out the liver and put in a stint to drain blockages in the liver.

I remember going to Neil's house that Monday morning. Our brother Hadley was there so we could pray together before we left. I know how bad it is from what I learned on the internet, but I keep it to myself. Prayer can change things, and I'm praying for that. That the test will show some mistake and all will be well. We're all praying for good news on this day.

I remember sitting in the waiting room with Mary while Neil is in having his procedure. We were also waiting for their son, Kenny, to arrive.

I can't tell Mary what I read on the internet. How could I? I asked her if she was prepared for the worst and she said, "I can't even imagine the worst." I have to wait to hear the doctor say it.

Kenny came to the hospital while Neil was in the procedure and waited with us. He was with us when we got the news.

I remember the nurse coming into the waiting room and telling us that the procedure was over and would we follow her so the doctor could talk with us. I think that was the longest walk I ever took. I knew it wasn't good when the doctor didn't come out himself. She showed us into an examining room where we waited a very short time for the doctor.

It was bad. The cancer was wrapped around the tubes that drain the liver. Doc said he had to put in two stints and that the cancer had spread from the pancreas to the liver. We sat there in shock while he told us Neil had six months to live! Oh God, Oh God, help us! How do you tell someone you love that they're dying?

Dr. B told us that with treatment he could possibly live for a year. I asked him about other treatments; you know the unconventional ones. After all, they admitted there was no cure, and maybe something else would work. He didn't really have an answer, so I asked him what he would do if it was his brother. He looked at me with such compassion and he really thought about it before he answered. I'm sure he was imagining it was his brother. After a thoughtful minute he said he would follow what the oncologist suggested.

Even though I was somewhat prepared, it was horrible hearing the words. Mary wept and I wept. Kenny sat quietly until the doc was finished and left. Then he fell apart, <u>totally.</u>

Kenny was devastated. He not only cried but he cried out, "NO, NO, not my Dad! NO not my Dad!" *We clung to each other in that little room and cried and tried to be strong for Kenny.* I remember telling him, "We have time Kenny. What if you'd just been told that Neil had died in an accident and was already gone. Kenny we have time. We have some time!"

Mary said she had to be the one to tell Neil. We pulled ourselves together as much as we could, and we left that little room. There was a waiting room right next to it and as we walked out, many eyes met ours and I knew they had heard us wailing. I remember thinking that any one of them or any of us could be only one doctor's appointment away from such news. There was a reality there that no one wanted to face. I also know that there were Christians there praying for us as we walked through. God is always there giving us what we need, when we need it.

Neil was admitted to the hospital and while Mary sat with him I made some phone calls. That was so hard. I had already called our brother Hadley, but did not reach him. I had to give the news to his son, who loved Neil very much. Well, we all did. Anyway, he was going to go tell his dad. I called our other brother, Keith, in California. We each clung to the phone receivers and cried for our brother and for ourselves because of our loss. And I called my husband and kids, and we cried. Mary and I later got a room at the hospital's connecting hotel.

The rest of the day we sat with Neil and waited. He was too groggy to tell, but he knew we were there and that it was bad. Later, when Mary and I went to our room before dinner we made some calls, had wine and talked. I'll never forget what she said, but I must write it down. She said, "I have been so blessed to have known this wonderful man and to have been loved by him. If anyone ever had a fairy tale marriage, it's me."

That had such an impact on me because it was so true. Neil and Mary were one. Truly, you never thought of one without the other. Best friends and companions that were always together. How could Mary go through this, lose Neil, and survive? God has promised that He will never allow more trials than we can handle. What is He thinking? How can any of us, especially Mary, survive this? I remember praying, "Lord, we trust You and love You, and if You say so, then it's true, we'll survive this, but You'll have to see us through every step of the way, but please, please heal Neil."

When faced with trials that you feel you cannot overcome or endure, please know that you can. You just have to keep pressing forward, one day at a time, and you will make it through. Mary is surviving this terrible loss in her life. She has to work hard at it, but she counts on the Lord to see her through, and He does, always by her side. It's a continuing process.

We cried, and prayed, and cried some more. Mary stayed with Neil by his bedside that night, and by the time I got there in the morning she had told him.

As I got ready the next morning in that hotel room, I was very anxious about seeing my brother. I was in a numb state of shock still. I remember walking down that hospital hallway thinking, "This can't be happening. I'm not really going in to see my brother who was just told he's dying. Lord please change this.......heal him". I felt like the things around me weren't real. The world had stopped.

It was hard to face the reality of it. Mary left us alone and Neil opened his arms for me to come to his bed, and he held me. We cried, hugged and told how much we loved each other. How unfair it was. How we'd all get through it together and it would be all right. And we just held onto each other tight, like we couldn't let go.

I remember asking Neil, "What am I going to do without you? We all need you in our lives. You've always been there for me." He said, "You've got Jed to take care of you and you've all got each other. You'll all be just fine." Much later I thought about this. Do you realize what I've just written? It was all about me.......what am I going to do without him? I felt selfish. Neil was just told he was dying of cancer and he was comforting me. So like him. That was one of those things I wish I could do over. Anyway, as we hung onto each other, and cried, I told him that I would not let him die. I simply wouldn't allow it. It wasn't going to happen. I would pray and pray for his healing and I would search and search until I found something that would cure him.

At that moment, I actually thought I had some control over the situation. It's so hard to reach the point when you realize that there are situations in your life that you have absolutely no control over. I think deep inside, I always knew I had no control over Neil's cancer, even though I wouldn't admit it. That's why I'd fall on my knees, and pray. Does God allow these things to happen to bring us to our knees to remind us of Him and His steadfast love? All I know is that His love was always present. His touch was always there. There was never a time that we blamed God, or turned away from Him. He was always our strength.

I can't help him. Oh God, I can't help him. Please do something. I had this overwhelming urge to call Mom and tell her Neil's in trouble and needs her. (She's in heaven.)
When Mary came back into the room, the three of us held hands and prayed.

Doc came in later and told Neil the facts, and possible treatments to give him more time. Neil listened, and told the doc he would do what he needed to do, in order to give him more time, but he was also concerned about his quality of life. Dr. B said the oncologist could answer his questions and help him decide what course to take. It was obvious Dr. B was sad for Neil and wished he had better news. *Neil, always cheerful and optimistic. As Dr. B was leaving the room, Neil said to him,*

"Hey doc, I've got a really bad headache. Could I get something for it? It's really killing me!" Ha Ha.
I'll never forget how Dr. B looked at him. That Neil actually used humor at such a time and tried to uplift the bearer of bad news. Doc definitely noticed and gently shook his head and grinned at Neil. He said, "Neil, I'll get you something for that, anything you want." I'm sure doc left there feeling not quite so bad. That's just the way Neil was. He had compassion for others.

That afternoon Neil's daughter, Tammy and her husband came in to see him. I remember I was sitting on the window sill, completely consumed by the situation. They came in full of smiles and exchanged pleasantries like you would if someone was just recuperating from a routine surgery. Then they pulled out a deck of cards and asked Neil to play cards with them. I was absolutely shocked. I couldn't believe it! This was the first time Tammy had seen her dad since finding out he was dying and she wanted to play cards! When they asked me to join, I declined and left the room. I needed some space. I wondered if I'd missed something here. Maybe it was just a bad dream after all, because when I returned, Neil was playing cards with them and being pleasantly normal.

You see, Neil in his compassion, saw something that I did not. He realized that Tammy, who loved her father very much, was not yet ready to accept his illness and impending death. She needed to grab hold of some normalcy. And so, Neil played cards with her and gave her what she needed at the time.
Later, she would take the time and words that only they would share.

When a family receives a blow like this one, you can expect different reactions. We each have our own self protection mechanisms. They're there to help us deal with a crisis at a pace that we can handle.

That day, Neil taught me a very important lesson in loving someone. It was a selfless love, unconditional. Not once through his entire illness did I hear him say, "What about me?" I hope I never have to find out if I could be so selfless. I'm afraid I would fall short.

4

Preparing For and Starting Treatment; Relying On Our Faith

Neil was released from the hospital the next day and soon after that he had his first appointment with Dr. J, the oncologist. Neil, Mary and I had discussed different possibilities in treatments, as I'm sure they discussed with themselves and their family. Neil didn't want to decide anything until he talked with Dr. J.

The morning of Neil's first appointment with the oncologist, Hadley came over to pray with us before we left. This became our routine as the months passed. Whenever Neil had to go in for an appointment, or a procedure, we always came together and prayed before we started our day. Praying for an easy day, guidance, good news, and always, always for healing. We never failed to pray for a miracle. His cancer was fatal, incurable. It would take a miracle from our Lord for him to be healed. We didn't care if that miracle came in the form of a new treatment, or if God just healed him in the blink of an eye. We just wanted him healed.

Oh how I prayed! It consumed me. Neil was constantly on my mind and I was constantly lifting him up in prayer. Sometimes it was just a little arrow prayer I would shoot up, but it was all the time. I'd fall asleep praying, and wake up in the night to pray, and start again in the morning.

I remember wondering once, if God had allowed this to happen so that we would all turn to Him completely, and rely on Him more. You'll notice I said 'allowed'. God didn't do this to us. It just happened. Probably from our own environment, since we are our own worst enemies. But He is Almighty God!! He could have stopped it or prevented it, but He didn't. I don't know the answer to that, but I know it did draw me closer to Him. Why wasn't I that close to Him before? Why was I always too busy? Regardless of the unanswered question, I do know that He was with Neil, and all of us, every second of this journey and long before and long after. He is forever, and always, with us. We are all His precious children.

Neil's appointment with Dr. J, the first of many, actually left us feeling like we could get a handle on this monster devouring his body, and have some control over it. We were excited, and hopeful, and really felt the touch of God and His hand on us. This entire journey was like a roller coaster. High and hopeful one minute, lost and devastated the next. Cancer in a family will cause enormous emotional turmoil. I don't know how non-Christians manage to get through. We totally relied on the Lord for strength and when we had none, He gave us something to bring us through and keep us going.

Neil's examination showed what good health he was in, excluding the cancer of course. Can you imagine! Dr. J wanted to put Neil into a test program that was trying different combinations of chemo to see if they would have a positive effect on pancreatic cancer. It wasn't so long ago that they didn't even make an attempt to battle pancreatic cancer. At least now they were trying, and Neil was healthy enough to be in the test program. The only problem was his liver had not yet bounced back from being clogged from the tumor. Once his liver count became closer to normal, he could start the program. Hurray!

He was having some problems before his chemo started, with high liver count and fevers. Can you imagine, his liver had cancer, but it needed to be healthier, before he started chemo. We prayed, (had been constantly since this started) and Neil started "juicing" fruits and vegetables to help his liver get better.

I kicked into action. My husband and I have a juicer and often make juice from vegetables for good health. I knew that beets were very good for the liver and blood. So, I gave Neil and Mary our juicer and the information about different vegetables and their benefits, and Neil started juicing it. Mary would make his juice every day. In the afternoon, Mary would put his beet juice in a wine glass, and they would have their glass of 'wine'. Would things ever be normal again?

April: Some time has passed and many emotions. Neil is so strong on the outside. He's always taking care of everyone else. And of course there is Nurse Ratchet, Neil's name for Mary. She takes such good care of him.

Neil had to go in for blood counts once a week, to see if his liver function was better, and finally we got the OK to start the new program. We were elated, and ready to start killing the monster.

Neil is so healthy that he was admitted into a new research program. How ironic is that! He's so healthy except that he's dying of cancer! Anyway, this new research uses two different chemo's that have been used before in pancreatic cancer separately, but never together. They've been perfected, and the research is that they'll use both of them at once. They will not cause nausea or hair loss. Neil has had two treatments so far, and this holds true. He feels fine. Remember how Neil was concerned about quality of life? This chemo doesn't sound like it will be too bad. This is a touch from God.

I remember when Neil had his first chemo treatment. I was with Neil and Mary when the nurses put the needle in him and pumped the chemo into his veins. Neil was such a cheerful patient, and the nurses loved him right off the bat. He spoke to all the other patients in the room and asked how they were doing. It was like doom and gloom in there, until Neil managed to bring everyone up a few notches. He'd sit in his chair and say, "Go to work chemo, kill, kill, kill. Zing! Wow, I felt that. It's dying. Zing! I can feel it dying." The other patients got a kick out of that.

When we got back to their home that afternoon my husband, Jed, came over and we decided to go out to dinner. Neil said he felt great, and I know he and Mary wanted something in their lives to be like it used to be. At dinner, Neil started shaking and was very cold. It was a very anxious meal, and we hurried through it, so we could get back home. Once there, we settled Neil into a warm nest, and took care of him.

I don't know what we were thinking. They had just pumped all that chemo into his system and we went out to dinner! We just wanted to do something normal. Normal, forget that. Once cancer hits, nothing is ever the same again. Your lives will be changed forever, and not only in the things you can or cannot do, but right down to the way you think and feel about things. It's amazing how fast your priorities change and you realize what is, and isn't important. I remember when Neil first found out he was dying. He said to me, "Hey, I don't have to sweat the small stuff anymore." He meant the everyday anxieties and problems we all face. Suddenly, they weren't such big problems!

After several treatments, Neil found that if he ate something light when he got home from chemo and went right to bed, he would feel better the next day. This became his routine on chemo days.

Neil was having problems with high fevers. The early bedtime on chemo days helped, but he just couldn't get over having the fevers, accompanied by chills. He wasn't so sick that he vomited, and he didn't lose his hair, but you can't have pancreatic cancer, receive chemo and have a good quality of life, as Neil found out. Mary and I both hurt so badly for him. He never complained, but we knew he didn't feel good. We'd ask him how he was, how he felt, and he always said, "fine". Then when we went to his doctor's appointments with him, we'd hear how he really felt! At least he was wise enough to tell his doctor! Still, he chose to stay on this path. It was the only medical hope he had.

Neil's liver count came down and he started his chemo, but still had a problem with fevers. More prayer. Hadley stood in for Neil one night at a prayer group and specifically prayed for Neil and the fevers. He hasn't had one since! The power of prayer is amazing and I cannot believe how many people all over this country are praying for my brother. Even people that don't know him.

Neil's fevers stopped! This was one more of those highs that I spoke about. One of those gifts from God when He lets you know He is with you and hears you. Oh, how we needed them. It never failed, whenever we were at our lowest, God would lift us up. When you're fighting a terminal cancer, the smallest of things can be monumental; good or bad.

5

Family, Friends & Prayer

I often tell my children, and grandchildren, that nothing is more important than family. Of course this does not include one's relationship with the Lord, which is foremost.

We may not always like a family member's personality or an act or statement they may have made, and we can be mad at them, but we must always love each other, take care of each other, and stand together as a family. Our family is like that. We've had our differences but we've never said harsh, unforgivable words. There have always been times when someone (all of us I'm sure) has been unlovable. Yet, we still love. That has always been one of those many blessings from God. (Besides, Mom always said we had to get along. Now I say it.)

Our whole family has always been blessed with good health. Now, we've all been devastated and we've all pulled together. That's what family is about. Hang onto that, stick together, and love one another. Be there for each other, so you can laugh together and cry together.

We all find ourselves being comforted by each other, and comforting each other right back. Hadley, Keith and I have comforted Neil and he has had to comfort us. Bless his heart. He is such a good man.

I am so thankful that by the grace of God, through His son Jesus, we are saved. How else would we find the strength for the battle ahead?

Back to the prayer. Power. That's what prayer is. And we have it. Many, many, are standing in prayer for Neil. Hadley makes a point of coming to Neil's on the mornings we leave for chemo; Neil goes once a week on Wednesdays; and the four of us pray. Of course we pray every day, but this is a special time.

We pray for healing, time, comfort, strength, and understanding. We pray for many things, all things. The doctors only hope to give Neil more time. I shouldn't say "only". I know his doctors, and I know it is their hope to find a cure, but they must be realistic. They love him already; the doctors, nurses, technicians. He's so optimistic and cheerful. He always wants everyone to have a wonderful day.

I know from Mary, and from Neil himself, that he has his sad times. Watching his grandchildren play, sitting in his back yard reflecting or spending time with all his loved ones. He cries. He wants to live, grow old with his wife, and watch his grandchildren grow.

You know, some people say it's God's will for some to die young. I don't believe that for one minute. God created us to live long and healthy lives. When God created man, he lived for hundreds and hundreds of years. We've poisoned our environment and our bodies, with chemicals and poor diets, and whatever else. God is not responsible for any of this. Man is his own worst enemy. I don't even know if you can blame Satan for it; even though he's glad we're so self destructive.

The Bible says we should thank God for all things. Mary and I have talked about this, and we can thank Him for the doctors, the research, the time given us, family, prayers, and all that comes about from this cancer. But we cannot thank Him for the cancer; for this happening to Neil. God has and will continue to bring good things from this, but we cannot thank Him for the cancer. I don't know how anyone could. I have since learned that this is not correct. The Bible actually says, in 1 Thessalonians 5:18, "*in* everything give thanks; for this is God's will for you in Christ Jesus"; not for all things, but in all things. This makes it much easier, for me, to understand and accept. As my pastor explained, "We give thanks that we are His and that we are in Him regardless of the circumstances."

Neil was now in a routine of receiving his chemo once a week. He didn't feel good but he and Mary tried to keep as normal a life as possible. The day we found out that he was dying, Mary and I quit his job for him. I guess no one took us seriously because Neil went to work, when he was able, just to check on things. He was the CEO of a business he and Hadley owned. He used to say he'd go in, see how business was, watch everyone cry because of his cancer, and then come back home. One day when I was at his home, Neil jokingly said he was going into work to make everyone cry, and then he'd be back. It didn't take long before he was back home! He wanted everyone to be comfortable with his cancer, and to get the initial shock out of their systems. This was very important to him, as I'm sure it is with most cancer patients. Please don't avoid someone because they are sick. They need to know that they are still the same people to you.

Neil was someone different to many people; husband, father, grandfather, brother, uncle, friend, boss. But no matter which person he was to others, they all loved him. Death is hard, and dying is harder. When put in a position like this, when someone you know is dying, it's so hard to know what to say or do. Because of this, many people won't do anything. They just continue on like nothing is wrong. I used to be the same way, but through this I've learned it's not a good thing to do. You need to say something to the person who's dying, or send them a card. Let them know that they matter to you and that you're thinking of them. It's important.

Neil got a lot of cards and phone calls. We have cousins in Reno who sent him a card every week. And they were so funny. I don't know where she found those cards, but Neil and Mary both looked forward to getting them. It's OK to be funny and it's so important to laugh.

I try to go with Neil and Mary every week to chemo. It's a long drive and an over night trip, but I need to be there, as much as they need me. We are definitely each other's support. When I'm home, I'm always praying and looking on the internet for something, anything, that we might use in our battle.

I can't sit by and let Neil die of cancer. I think, for a very short time, I thought he would get better and this chemo would kill all the cancer. I realized that although I want that to happen, the doctors have never changed their prognosis. Time. They are only giving us some time. I pray and pray for an answer. I'm afraid the time will come when they say the chemo has stopped being effective and they can do no more.

We must have a plan B for when that happens. I found a book called "A Cancer Battle Plan" by Anne Frahm and her husband. She was a "hopeless" case sent home to die. She turned to nutritional healing treatment and was soon cancer free. For now, until we find something better, this will be our Plan B.

Neil already is incorporating nutrition into Plan A (the chemo). He knows he must heal his liver. The liver cleans and purifies the blood. It's essential to good health.

As the chemo kills everything in his body, he must replace the nutrients. I'll gladly grasp this straw of hope.

It's strange when you are faced with such a situation, how the least little positive thing is so much; when you have nothing else but hope, and you're told it is hopeless. I will never give up the fight for Neil's life.

I've decided I don't like the word "hopeless". It goes against the very meaning of the word hope. To say there is no hope is to say the word doesn't exist. There is always hope. Things may not end the way we want them to, but there is always hope…always!

Thank you Lord for Your many blessings. For the strength you give us; for family and friends, for doctors and research in every area, including nutrition. Thank you for salvation and thank you for hope!

6

Mary's Strength From God

Let me tell you something about Neil's wife Mary. I've known her for many years, but through this nightmare I learned what a remarkable woman she is. As I said before, Neil and Mary make up one unit. The other half of her was sick and dying. Her life had changed forever without any warning. She wanted to be the one to take care of Neil and his every need and she wanted to be with him all the time. She took control from the start and just stepped right into the task at hand. When he started his chemo, because it was a research program, it came with a lot of paperwork. Everything had to be documented, and right from the beginning Neil had many different medications to take. He had a couple of different pain pills, long acting and short term, which he had to take at different times of the day. Since these caused constipation, he also had pills to help with that and sleeping pills, anxiety pills, and pills for nausea, and so on and so on. It was too much to remember, so she used a chart to help her remember what medications needed to be taken when. She made sure everything was done on time and documented.

This may not sound like a great task, but know this….you cannot even imagine the stress of fighting for the life of a loved one when the doctors give you no hope, until you've experienced it. Neil was my brother and I was beside myself with grief and fear of the unknown yet to come. Neil was Mary's husband. He was a major part of her and so a part of her was dying too. She lived with him and in a 24-hour day she saw all his hopes, dreams, agony, pain and fear of what lay ahead for them. When Neil hurt, she also hurt for him. She was unable to protect him and help him get better. She just had to ride the wave. She was in a nightmare situation that she had no control over. As she dealt daily with this battle, she was under a tremendous amount of stress. So much so that even the smallest things sometimes seemed like mountains. Yet, she prevailed. She and Neil had such faith in God that they knew He was with them and they would make it through this. And as Mary told me many times, she often questioned God and tried to convince Him that she couldn't do it. But He kept giving her the strength she needed. He gave all of us what we needed to get through this.

We have a large family and many friends. When we would return from a doctor's appointment, or a procedure, Neil and Mary's answering machine would be full of messages. Everyone wanted and needed an update on how he was doing. It became overwhelming for Mary to find the time to make all those phone calls, but she did the best she could.

In order to help Mary with this task, Hadley decided to start sending out emails once a week or so to give everyone updates on Neil's progress. This began the 'Neil Updates' that everyone looked forward to. I will also incorporate the 'Neil Updates' into my writing.

7

Waiting for Results and Visitations

June: It's been too long since I've written in here. Sometimes I just need to keep to myself and it's just hard to take the time.

As Neil progressed with his chemo and his juicing he felt very encouraged and hopeful, yet uncertain if it was working. After chemo he didn't get physically sick, but would get high fevers and severe chills. We of course, prayed for him and now that doesn't happen anymore. He finds that on the day of chemo, if he comes home and goes straight to bed for a long nap he feels much better.

During those first weeks of chemo and juicing, we had no idea what was happening to Neil's liver and pancreas. The Dr. wouldn't do another scan until he'd finished a full series of chemo, which was six weeks. It was hard waiting to find out if things were getting better or worse. This was a difficult time for us, and we prayed that God would let us know. We needed a sign.

The end of April Neil felt tired and went to bed early but couldn't sleep. As he lay in bed, two nurses appeared beside the bed. Now, Neil was shocked! At first he thought he was dreaming except he knew he wasn't asleep and when he was sure he was awake he thought he was hallucinating. When the nurses spoke to him he knew they were real. They spoke clearly and said, "The Lord is sending two warriors to help you fight your battle." And they were gone.

Neil said he just lay there unable to really move or call to Mary because he was so shocked. I think he was under the power of the Holy Spirit. As he lay there, he could sense, not actually see, but sense two angels, warriors, in the room with him, and Neil also knew that they were holding spears!

As he slept and woke through the night he could feel their presence and he kept telling Mary about the two warriors fighting for him. In the morning he told her about the nurses and warriors, and then she understood his night time rambling about warriors!

Neil had an appointment the day after this visitation, and when Hadley and I were there to pray, he told us about it. I can't tell you how much we need a sign from God. Sometimes when you pray and pray, and you're in agony and grief, it starts to weigh heavy on your heart and mind and you wonder if it's getting through. I know I did. We never felt discouraged from praying, but we sure did need some sign. We knew the Lord heard our prayers and that He was with us, because He always did little things to make our day easier, but we needed a big sign, a real statement that said, "Yes I hear you and I'm on it." Well, when we heard Neil's story we all had goose bumps big time. I was just in awe....wow! OK, OK we've really got help now!

Do I believe this was a divine visitation? ABSOLUTELY!! Visitations are recorded throughout the scriptures. Our Lord is so wonderful, He knew Neil, all of us, needed to know we aren't alone in this.

Actually, there have been other visitations in our family. Probably more than I know about. I remember many years ago when I was a new Christian and very earnest in praying for my father's salvation. I would pray and pray for him, that his heart would soften to the Lord so he could see and understand the salvation awaiting him as a gift. I would actually cry and plead and fast and pray to the Lord. On one such day, I was alone in my bedroom crying and praying for my father and a dove appeared above the bedroom door. It wasn't that I could actually reach out and touch it, but it was there. Beautiful white and glowing. I just knelt there staring at it and I felt washed and flooded by God's spirit. It was wonderful. This gave me the reassurance that my father would accept salvation, but it didn't mean for me to stop praying for him. I continued to pray, but I wasn't praying with such anguish. You see, I had previously witnessed to my dad and shared salvation with him. I asked if he wanted to accept Christ as his savior and he very politely said, "Thank you honey, but I'm not ready to do that." So I was anguished when I prayed and I was afraid for him. Even after this vision of the dove, my father did not become a Christian for several years! Dad quietly gathered the seeds we all gave him and God slowly nurtured them until one day dad announced he was getting baptized.

The other visitation was to my mother. Now, I want you to understand that my parents were not 'godly straight and narrow' people. They were socializing party people. They had lots of friends and had lots of parties. Mom was Catholic and had a strong faith and loved God, but she never had that __personal__ understanding of salvation. Even though she went to church every Sunday and prayed every day, she actually was born again after dad, and that was when they were both in their seventies!

I remember sitting in the office at work. We were alone and the Holy Spirit put it on my heart to talk with her about salvation, which I did. She started crying and said she didn't think anyone was ever going to ask her! Hadley came into the office to find us both crying.

Her visitation came while on her death bed. She had stopped eating and taking fluids and we knew she was ready to go home to be with the Lord soon. I was alone with her one afternoon and she was very weak and it was difficult for her to talk. She kept staring around her bed and raised her hand to touch something. After she did this a couple of times, I asked what it was, did she see something? She nodded her head and raised her hand out again. I asked her what she saw and she said, "Angels!" My mother saw the angels around her bed, to give her comfort and to take her home! I so wanted to see them too, but this was just for her. I was so thankful that she was able to share that with me.

Some may think these were all brought on by stress, emotion or whatever, but if you know God, you know they were not. I truly believe in God's presence and His touch. And I believe these were all from Him.

When I was told about Neil's angels, I was so thankful, but at the same time the Lord pointed out to me, in that quiet voice where He speaks inside your head, that the warriors were there to help him 'fight his battle'. He didn't say 'win'. (I won't share this with anyone.)

Remember, that this is from my journals. When God pointed this out to me, I had to stand back. What, what do you mean, fight but not win; fight not win? But that was all I got, and it was enough for me to know Neil may not survive this terminal cancer. This was the first time that God was letting me know Neil wasn't going to make it. Where was our miracle? There was no way I was going to share that with anyone. I knew we needed the hope and encouragement that the message of the warriors brought. But God knew I was headed for a terrible blow because I truly, truly believed Neil would get well. He was gently and slowly preparing me.

Neil's angels gave him the encouragement he needed, but it was obvious it was going to be a "battle". His treatment is like a roller coaster, up and down with good days and bad. But we are not alone!!

Neil Update 5/12/00: Hi folks. Would have written last week but it was Neil's off week for chemo and he had a few good days off. This week was his double dose week with the regular chemo and the experimental one. The doctor's report was good; his blood count was better than the week before as was his liver. He even gained a little more weight. The "love handles" have come back. The day after chemo, Thursday, Neil stayed home and rested. Last night he got the shakes, like he was really cold and they would not stop. Mary started to rub him down and they asked the angels, through our Lord Jesus Christ, to help them. Soon the shakes went away and Neil also received a good night's sleep. Thank you Jesus for your great love for Neil and Mary and how you respond in his need. PLEASE ALL OF YOU, keep praying for him. God is there to help, but He wants us to ask and to keep asking! In two weeks, Neil will receive another cat scan to learn the effect of the chemo on the liver and the tumors.
Please say hello to all your family from us. Look forward to seeing you again. Stay healthy and in love with our Redeemer. With our love, Hadley and Peggy Psalms 90:12 and 91:11 God Bless You.

8

Siblings Retreat & Prayer

As Neil's treatments progressed and he and Mary tried to adjust to the changed life that cancer brings, he battled depression and wanted more than anything to enjoy life the way he used to. He was still sad about missing his trip to Chili and the Panama Canal. Travel was hard to plan with his chemo treatments but they really wanted to go somewhere to escape reality as much as possible, even for a few days. His chemo was once a week for three weeks, but the week off he still had to go in for a blood test. We decided to all go to Palm Springs to visit our brother Keith. The doctor arranged for Neil to have his blood test a few of days early and this gave us a couple of extra days. We went all out; got a limo to the airport and Neil and Mary were able to score an upgrade for the only two extra seats available in first class. That was one thing Neil always managed to get, great upgrades.

We went to Palm Springs in May. We were there less than a week, five days I think, but it was so good to all be together for the first time since Neil was diagnosed. Neil was very ill the first day, but got better. The pain pills cause terrible constipation so he has to take meds to counter that.

Palm Springs was very good for all of us. The first day was rough because Neil was so sick, and although it made us very aware of the gravity of the situation, it was so wonderful for us siblings to be together, and stand with Neil in prayer, and to petition for that miracle healing we needed. We joined in prayer every day and that was such a special time to be together and feel God's presence. We also had prayer for Neil at Keith's church. The cancer never left my mind.

Keith's wife, Nancy, treated us like royalty and was truly a wonderful hostess. We felt like we'd come off a battle field, anyway I did, and she just took care of us. It was so needed and so appreciated. We had so much fun just playing together like kids and teasing at one another.

Keith took us out shooting one day; yes guns. Just the four of us went, me and my three brothers, which made it all the more special. We all practiced and then Keith put up some targets. Neil got a bull's eye. I remember how exciting that was at first and then how much it bothered me. I felt uncomfortable about it. I was thinking, "Why did he get that; because he won't live to get another chance at one?" I would sometimes get these little flames of anger shooting out of me, because I really was angry about the whole thing. Anger is natural in cancer, and healthy, as long as you understand it. Was this a natural anger toward God or was I just angry? Cancer is so unfair, and dying young is not right. Even though I was angry, I was never too angry to pray. Prayer was all that kept me going. I don't believe I was angry at God, because I understood He was not responsible, and although He might not change it, I was able to leave it in His hands, regardless of the outcome.

Neil Update 5/22/00: This is our 6th and last day with Keith and Nancy at their wonderful home in Palm Springs. The weather has been a bit hot, but still great! Peggy and I are here with Gaynel, Neil and Mary, and of course our hosts Keith and Nancy.

Hi, this is Gaynel. It's more than a bit hot, 106!! We are having such a good time together. Lots of laughs and good, good food. Nancy sure can cook. My brothers seem to think they should try to drown me in the pool. Some great water fights, but I can hold my own. Neil had a rough day the first day here, but soon felt better. We pray together daily and lay hands on him. Yesterday at church we did the same at Keith's bible study. Neil seems to be in a bit more pain, but we won't give up the fight! Wednesday he has another CT, so we'll see the results of the chemo. We will hopefully start also working with a nutritionist who will work with the oncologist. We have to try everything, everything, everything!!

Hi, this is Neil now. Having a great time; wonderful food, great family, wonderful prayer. Too damn hot!!

9

The First Cat Scan; God Heard Our Prayers

We were looking forward to getting back from Palm Springs only because Neil was scheduled to have his first CT Scan since he'd started the research treatment program. We had no idea what was happening in there, just that the blood tests looked better. Neil was the first patient to begin the program and his doctor was sharing his progress with the other pancreatic cancer patients. They were all looking to Neil, hoping for good results.

Another trip into Seattle to the hospital clinic, turning the car over to the valet parking, into the building and up the elevator and through the halls to the x-ray, sign in and wait for Neil to be called. We'd done this before and would do it many, many times more before this journey ended. I remember when I was sitting in the waiting room, I'd look around at the other people waiting for their tests, and I'd wonder what was on their plate. Was it something as simple as ulcers, or as devastating as terminal disease? They didn't know my brother was dying. I didn't know if any of them were dying. I'd pray for Neil and good test results and his healing and I'd shoot up a prayer for everyone there. I'm sure there were others there praying also.

We always had to wait after Neil had his tests. They had to be read by the x-ray doctor and then sent to his oncologist. Usually a trip to the hospital clinic took all day with tests in the morning and the doctor appointment in the afternoon. This particular day was very long. We couldn't wait to find out the results.

May 24, 2000: *When we got back, Neil's first CT since he started chemo showed that all the tumors in his liver had shrunk and many had disappeared!!! The tumor in the* *pancreas was perhaps a little smaller but certainly not worse. This had us <u>elated</u>!! Finally some good news!*

Neil Update 5/24: Just heard from Gaynel who is with Neil and Mary at the hospital. They received the doctor's report from the cat scan taken earlier today. Neil's pancreas shows no change, meaning not worse! His liver shows that some of the cancer spots have disappeared and all the others are shrinking! PRAISE THE LORD FOR HIS MERCY!! The only problem was that the bile was beginning to back up again into the liver instead of draining. They said this was most likely due to a blocked stint and they can replace it with a new one. So right now Neil and Mary are a couple of happy campers. That's all for now; hope to hear from you. Have a great holiday weekend. We love you, Hadley and Peggy.

Oh, I just can't tell you how happy we were after that news. We had the cancer on the run; it was being killed and the tumors were shrinking! The doctor was very pleased but he was still reserved and said we'd have to wait and see. We didn't let that discourage us though and we felt like celebrating! We were on a high again that lasted less than two weeks.

Then he had a setback. His bilirubin count was up in his liver, meaning the stints were blocked and had to be replaced. Another procedure!

Neil Update June 8, 2000: Neil had surgery yesterday to replace the stints in his liver because the old ones had plugged. The new ones are in and the liver is draining again just the way it's supposed to. The doctor also told him his liver is continuing to improve. The cancer tumors are still disappearing! Also, the tumor on the pancreas is getting smaller. Neil's strength is returning and the pain is less. He is indeed one of the thousands. He comes home from the hospital today. Please keep praying. Hadley and Peggy.

Dr. B, the doctor that did the first scope on Neil and found the cancer and put in the first stints, is the one that replaced them. He was very surprised at how much better everything looked and pleased with Neil's progress. This was more good news and another high for us. We give all the glory to God and continue to pray for healing.

He's felt better since the new stints but the pain is still there, which brings us to the present pain block, pray it works!!

With the liver draining properly, Neil felt much better, but the pain was getting worse. I don't understand this and it is really a concern for me. If the tumors are shrinking, why is the pain getting worse? Neil doesn't stand straight, leaning to his right side. Why? This should be improving too, shouldn't it? I'm so afraid and so full of unanswered questions. We are anxiously waiting for the next CT.

June 2000: Neil continues with his treatment. He seems to feel good. He looks good too, but I can tell he's not. Mary says he has more bad days than good, and he stands leaning to his right side; he favors the side where the pain is. He tires easily and he fights the blues. The last two days (26th & 27th) they did a pain block for him in his spine. Hopefully it will last a full year but they say it could only last two months. He wants so badly to get off most of the pain pills. It is so discouraging that the cancer is receding but the pain is not.

Neil Update July 18, 2000: Dear family and friends: Neil called me this afternoon after he returned from the hospital, with good news. His blood test showed that his "tumor markers" (a measure of tumor growth I think) had gone from 52,000 at the time of the doctors discovering his cancer to 12,000 today! A remarkable turnaround. The doctor was very happy, not to mention Neil and Mary.
This is not the most exact of tests, but a week from tomorrow Neil will receive a cat scan which will show exactly the retreat of the cancer. I will certainly write you again on that date.
Thank you very much for your continued prayers. For some reason, the Lord is truly listening and acting on our request for a healing in Neil's body. Please keep praying! With love and thanks, Hadley and Peggy

I think with Neil's first CT showing the improvement of the tumors and his blood tests showing a drop in the tumor marker, we relaxed a bit in our efforts. I know Neil was very tired of the juices he had to drink a couple of times a day and he backed off on them. I'm sure a lot of people thought he was going to beat the unbeatable cancer. I wrote in my journal: *I'm so happy and hopeful. The chemo is working; please God let this be the beginning of total healing.* The doctor had also remarked at how the others in the research program were so excited about Neil's reports. Another high.

10

The Chemotherapy Routine; Putting Things Into Perspective

I go with Neil and Mary to his chemo treatments as often as I can. It's incredible how one whole floor of the hospital is just for patients to receive chemo. Neil goes once a week, but some have to go every day. It's hard for me to do, but I have to remember how much harder it is for him and for Mary. I don't like that he has to go through this. Please God, let this be Your vessel for healing him. It's so hard to watch the 'needle work'. They always have to find a healthy vein to poke. I know the chemo is poison, killing good with bad, but it's all we have.

Neil's attitude is always good. He loves to tease his nurses and be happy with the other patients. Always a happy man on the outside. When he gets his chemo he says, "Kill, kill, kill that cancer. Zap, I can feel them dying."

I remember how the nurses enjoyed Neil and how the other patients seemed to lighten up a bit when he was there. He always seemed to do that, bring people around him up a level, even in that place. I almost said 'that sad place', but it would really be sad if you didn't have the option of chemo and the chance to beat it and live. It was a hard place to be, but we were glad it was there.

Neil Update July 29, 2000: On Tuesday I went to the hospital with Neil, Mary and Gaynel. We spent the day going through the procedures that Neil encounters every week. We arrived before 8:00 and went to the 4th floor for Neil to have his blood drawn for tests. After that he went in for a cat scan that was on the same floor. By this time it was about 10:30, so we went down stairs to the lunch room for something to eat. About noon, we went up to the 12th floor to check in for chemo and then the doctor visit. The conference with the doctor and Neil's regular nurse was very interesting. They were both very pleasant and up front in answering our questions. The cat scan showed no change from the last time, which was disappointing to us, as we expected a great improvement in his condition. They both assured us it was still good news. There is no growth of the cancer. It is stopped. The large tumor on the pancreas could possibly be scar tissue that will always be there, or the tumor could still be alive and become active if the treatments were stopped. Gaynel of course was asking the questions, and they were being answered very well. After the doctor interview we went into the infusion room where Neil would receive his chemo. It was an hour wait for the chemo to arrive so time was spent talking, reading and walking around. The room was a medium size hospital room with five chairs that reclined. Each chair had a patient waiting or receiving chemo. It was quite crowded, especially with we three extras. But no one minded us being there. While waiting, I walked the hall looking into all the rooms. Each was the same, five chairs, five chemo patients. It starts early in the morning and goes on all day. Hundreds every day, receiving chemo, and hundreds more in the basement taking radiation for cancer. And this is just one hospital! The number of people just in Seattle fighting for their lives against cancer was overwhelming to me. And so many who seemed to have no hope. Also while waiting, I read a report on survival rates of five years on the major types of cancer. Pancreatic cancer, 46,300 cases a year, had a 4% survival rate for five years. That was by far the worst. All the others were between 40% and 96%. Neil is one of the 4%, and we are certainly asking the Lord for more than five.

After Neil's chemo, we were done for the day and headed home. It was a day I will not soon forget. Neil goes through this every week and after one visit I didn't want to go back. Well, I've said enough, love you all, Hadley.

Hadley's one day in Neil's life at the hospital was a real eye opener for him. Most people aren't aware of what is going on in our hospitals; how many people are battling cancer and fighting for their lives. I know for me it has changed how I look at things in my own life. Ever since Neil was diagnosed, my priorities changed dramatically. I can't even remember what some of them were.

It definitely changed my attitude about my fibromyalgia. The winter before Neil's diagnosis had been a hard one for me. I ached and hurt every day, as you do with fibro, and I was into a few pity parties. When Neil got sick, I switched gears very quickly. Nothing about me mattered; I only thought about Neil. So what if I had an ache, at least it wasn't killing me and never would. There were many days that I never even thought about it. Even now I feel very fortunate that I have nonthreatening fibro and not cancer. It's amazing how, when we concentrate on others, we feel so much better ourselves. There is a lesson to be learned in that; like it's better to give than receive. No matter how bad things seem, they could be worse. Remember that. Even as bad as things were for Neil, it could have been worse.

I remember one incident when someone was complaining to me about how their neck ached. This person knew what I was going through with my brother's battle and they were complaining to me about a stiff neck. I wanted to slap them up along side the head! Forgive me again Lord, here was another one of those instances when my anger was poking out. I found that I did not have a great deal of patience during this time. I guess now, looking back, I didn't understand how other people's lives could go on as normal when mine had stopped. This journey definitely brought out every possible emotion in all of us, and the stress we were under had its effects.

11

Stress & Fear; The Second Cat Scan

Neil Update Aug. 1, 2000: Just a short note this time and a request. When I had prayer with Neil and Mary this morning before they left for the hospital, it became clear to me that they needed encouragement. Please forward this to your family and ask them also to send a card. Mary is sick with a cold (Neil had to take her to the doctor!) She can't get to close to Neil for fear of infecting him. His immune system is weak and the last thing he needs is another thing to fight. Also, Neil is beginning to realize that this struggle is for a long time. He is a bit down with that and the constant pain, though a lot less. It helps for us to cry and pray and lean on our Lord Jesus Christ. Please continue to pray and send encouragement. Hadley

I suppose it was inevitable for Mary to get sick. The stress she is under has to be lowering her immune system and this just adds to the stress! Now she has to worry about Neil getting sick.

Mary is sick with a cold and all she and any of us can think about is Neil's safety. His immune system is low. Lord, please make Mary better, and protect Neil. I know they are discouraged that their lives have changed so totally. Nothing is the same; everything revolves around the cancer. For me too. I pray constantly while I go about my day. I worry about my brother all the time.

Being a Christian doesn't mean you won't be afraid, it just means you don't have to fear death. Mary has told me how afraid she and Neil are. I know I'm afraid. She said they cry together, and hold on tight, and pray together, often. She said Neil was sitting in the back yard by himself one day, and when she checked on him he was crying. He's so tired of the fight and the pain, but he wants to live. The discouragement is difficult to overcome, because every time we get good news, we seem to get knocked back down. And even with the good reports, Neil doesn't feel good and is still in pain.

Neil has to go in for another CT and we are very happy about it and very anxious to see the results. We have been praying and praying for good results, and after the last CT we're hoping the liver tumors are all gone.

Neil Update Sept. 8, 2000: It's been over a month since my last update. Where did the time go? The whole summer seemed to go very fast. We sure feel fall weather here now. All of us, Neil, Mary, Keith, Nancy, Jed, Gaynel, Hadley and Peggy have decided to get together in Reno in October. We will visit our cousins who live there and it will be a very good time.

We're not sure of Neil's progress at this point. He's feeling better and has gained weight and has some control of the pain. Also the six months the doctors gave him is about up and he's looking at two years and beyond. When he went into the hospital Tuesday for chemo and a CT, the scan machine broke after showing the lungs and pancreas, so they did not get to see the liver. The pancreas looked the same, but one lung showed a small amount of fluid in the lower lining. Dr. J said it wasn't anything that concerned him, "just a bit of fluid". The doctor also said that Neil's tumor marker tests are not a good scale for how things are going because the markers are going up and down so much that he can't figure out why. So pray for stability in this test.

Early this morning, Neil had to go back into the hospital to have his liver stints replaced, as the old ones were beginning to plug. He will have to spend the night there. Mary and Gaynel are both with him of course. The doctor should get a good look at the liver while he's in there so we'll let you know how it turns out. The next week he's back in for chemo on Tuesday and a cat scan again on Friday.

The fight continues, but our Lord Jesus is faithful and full of mercy. He will carry Neil and Mary through this.

Please continue to pray for them as the emotional battle is just as hard as any. They need cards of encouragement and phone calls. They appreciate every one of you and speak often of all the prayers going before our Redeemer on their behalf. May our Lord richly bless each of you. Hadley

Neil Update: Sept. 8, 2000. Neil had his surgery yesterday to replace the stints in his liver so it could drain properly. All went very well. One of the old stints had dropped and was poking into an intestine so the doctor was glad to get it out before it caused damage. The liver is doing very well. Neil's operation went so well they sent him home the same day.

The doctors are calling Neil the Virginia Mason Poster Boy! Now that is a hard one to believe! We are all very happy and relieved to see Neil recovering so well.
Please keep he and Mary in your prayers, as the cancer is still there until who knows when? God knows, and He will tell us when to stop lifting Neil in prayer. Our God is an awesome God, worthy of all our praise and worship. Amen. We love you, Hadley

Journal: *Neil's stint replacement went so well they sent him home the same day. One of them had dropped down, hopefully now he won't be in such pain. I hate that; I can tell he hurts even if he doesn't complain. We are so hopeful!*

One of the many things Neil taught me through this by his own example was: You can be in pain without being a pain. Mary said he never complained and he never did to me. Every time we'd go to his doctors appointments we'd find out how he was really feeling; you know when they do that 'on a one to ten scale where is your pain'. Mary and I were always surprised by his answer and how much pain he was in, because he never told us. He said he did it to protect himself from us because we always tended to over do it when it came to taking care of him. Poor man, he was so patient with us.

12

There Is No Escaping Cancer

The winter before Neil found out he was sick, he came up with a great idea for we four siblings and spouses. He suggested that once a year we take a short trip together for a long weekend or even a week. It would just be the eight of us getting together, having fun and drawing closer together as a family. We decided we would take turns each year picking out where to go and we were all looking forward to it. Neil said he would choose the first year, but we were all thinking about where or what we would choose for our turn. What fun! We were looking forward to years of these great little trips. I decided I was going choose a dude ranch and ride horses when it was my turn. Someone else said something about going to San Francisco for a long weekend. We were all making plans into the future. Little did we know that after that one doctor's appointment in March we would only have time for one trip.

Neil made all the plans and reservations. We arrived separately at the hotel resort in Reno and it was so fun to wait for each other and get together. This trip was a little respite from the cancer routine. Neil had reservations for us in the 'black tie' restaurant. We had a private dining room and a wonderful meal and all of us dressed to the hilt like we didn't have a care in the world.
The next day, Neil had arranged for a limo to take us around Lake Tahoe, sight seeing and stopping for lunch. We also had a good visit with our cousins. We were away from the reality of cancer and the pressures of the battle if only for a short time.

We siblings and spouses went to Reno for a long weekend planned by Neil. We had such a great time just being together. I know Neil didn't feel good and he tired easily; what a trooper he was. Neil has chemo for three weeks and then one week off. We went during his week off because he tends to feel better then. (But not much) Oh Lord, I wish I could help him. Please let me help him.

The doctors are pleased with him; he seems to be making progress in a cancer that only kills.

As nice as it was to get away and be together, it didn't make any difference in the reality of the cancer. It came with us. There was no escaping it even though we were on another high while in Reno. Things supposedly were looking good for Neil and we were away on a fun trip, but it was always in the background, lurking like a thick dense fog ready to consume us. Oh Lord, will this nightmare ever end and Neil be well?

We returned home and the routine continued as always. Neil had a cat scan scheduled for the end of the month and we were praying for great results. I prayed constantly and was sure we would see a miracle. God, how much suffering must Neil endure before he can bear witness of Your mighty miracle? I kept thinking, how will anyone know it's a miracle if Neil isn't really bad? Please Lord, do something soon, I can't stand to see him hurt.

Every time we would return from one of Neil's procedures, Hadley would call me to get the details for his emails. To save time and the possibility of error I started doing the emails myself. Actually I found it to be a great form of therapy for me. It helped so much to give the details and especially to ask for help. I looked forward to it and often worried that I'd taken something from Hadley that was helpful to him. Writing things down has always been good for me, hence this story of our journey. It's helping me heal.

13

Changing Treatment & The Decline; Lord Please Help Us

The end of October 2000 marks seven months since Neil's diagnosis, and the beginning of the end. The worst was yet to come and it was an awful ride with one hurdle after another.

Neil was very tired and having trouble breathing. Well, not really trouble breathing, he was just short of breath and couldn't seem to get a full breath. We were looking forward to his upcoming appointment.

Neil Update October 31, 2000: I went with Neil and Mary yesterday for his six-week cat scan. Of course we prayed for more shrinkage of the tumors and continued healing. Dr. J told us that one more of the tumors in the liver had indeed shrunk. However, the small amount of fluid that was found in the last CT in Neil's lower right lung had increased. This was why he couldn't get a full breath. There was too much fluid taking up lung space.

Dr. J referred to it as "sympathetic infusion". He said there was a 50/50 chance that it could be cancerous. An appointment was made to have a procedure done to remove the fluid and have it tested. Before we even had time to pray for an appointment as soon as we could get one, the special research nurse on Neil's case got one for that very afternoon! Here was yet another touch from God. They removed most, if not all of the fluid, and the doctor doing the procedure said it was clear, and clear was good. However, we will not have the results of the test until Thursday. Our prayer request is as always, for continued healing, but specifically now for the fluid to be benign. Our Lord's hand is so strong in all of this and He is so good. He told Neil at the beginning that he was in a battle, and it truly is. Satan is always there, it seems, to jab at us with negatives, especially when we see God's touch. We have to constantly come against him and the discouragement he brings and pray for God's protection. We praise God for His faithfulness and His grace. Gaynel

Neil Update Nov. 1, 2000: Our news today was not good. The fluid in Neil's lung was very high protein, a precursor to cancer cells. It is good news that this was found before it actually became cancerous cells. What happens now is our concern. Neil will be taken out of the research program he is in, since it is obviously not effective. (It's strange how it is working in the liver and pancreas yet it is spreading somewhere else.) He will be placed in another research program to try a different chemo. How do we pray now? God is all powerful and He knows Neil's (and Mary's) needs. I pray that; 1. He doesn't have to wait too long before starting a new treatment, giving the cancer a chance to grow stronger. 2. The new treatment is effective and brings recovery and healing to him. 3. The new chemo does not make him sick, or his hair fall out. 4. That he only has to go to the hospital once a week for treatment. These last two seem like luxuries in the realm of it all, but I don't want him sick, or discouraged, or to have to go through any of this. I want my brother healed. I pray for God's continued healing, His touch, strength, and encouragement for Neil and Mary. "And we know that in all things God works for the good of those who love Him, who have been called according to His purpose." Romans 8:28. Neil and Mary surely do love Him <u>and trust Him in all things.</u> We don't know what His purpose is or what the 'good' will be, but wouldn't it be nice if through this agony, Neil's case and research was the one that found the cure! Please pray for healing, encouragement and protection. And pray that the Holy Spirit will bring Neil to people's minds as they are praying so he is not forgotten at prayer time. Gaynel

Journal: Neil has to go off his test chemo. The fluid in his lung got worse and it showed it was high protein, meaning it would turn to cancer. I'm so scared. How long will he have to wait before he can start another chemo and will the cancer grow fast in the meantime? GOD HELP US!

When Dr. J told us that Neil had to go off the research chemo he was on we were so disappointed. Neil was so upset and discouraged about this news of stopping the research program that he made a comment to Dr. J that I will never forget because it bothered me so much. It was the only time I saw Neil show his anger or any bit of defeat. After being told he had to stop the research program, he said, "So what am I suppose to do now, bend over and kiss my ass good bye?" I remember letting out a small cry of anguish, not because of what he said, but because he sounded so defeated. I just wanted to hold him and make it all go away.

All we knew to do was whatever the doctor told us. Many times in the following months, Mary told me, she wished they had insisted that Neil be left in that treatment program at least until we knew for sure what was happening with his lung. We always felt that once he stopped that chemo, which was gemcitabine, the cancer got control again. I know the doctors know so much more than we do since they see this every day, but it's something we will always look back on and wonder about. Don't be afraid to push a point with your doctor until you're satisfied with the answer.

The most frightening part of this step from one chemo program to the next was the time between. Neil had to wait a few weeks between and we knew we were dropping our defenses. There was nothing there to fight the cancer.
We were solemn to say the least. As part of our little support system, I always tried to be positive and look at the bright side. I told them, "Hey, this is just a bump in the road. The next chemo may be the best yet; the one to stop the killer."
We'd already had a lot of "bumps in the road" and as time went on, I had to quit saying it. There were just too many.

During the weeks we had to wait, Neil didn't feel good enough to travel too much. His favorite place was the 'beach house', their vacation home at the ocean, so he and Mary went there quite a bit and Neil did what he could to keep the battle going by giving his body what it needed in nutrients, by having his juice drinks and vitamins.

They were supposed to go to Eastern Washington for Thanksgiving, but Neil said he didn't feel good enough to go for the two plus hour drive, and spend the night. Unfortunately, his kids and their families had already gone so they missed spending that holiday with him. But it was fortunate for me and my family because we were getting together at my daughter's home and she lives in the same town as Neil and Mary, so they came over and we all had a very special day with them. Neil put up a good front, but I could tell he did not feel well at all. I have a picture of him on my desk that was taken that day and he looks so good. That was what everyone always said through his entire illness. "He looks so good." Up until the last couple of months, Neil did not look sick, with the exception of the way he leaned to his right side.

Neil Update: Nov. 25, 2000: Neil had to have a physical Thursday Nov. 16 before he could start a new chemo research program. His leg was in a great deal of pain. He thought it was a flare up of gout, but they discovered a blood clot behind his knee. Mary has to give him shots in his stomach twice a day for a short while, plus he's on a blood thinner. More pills. Evidently blood clots are common in chemo patients and now that he's on blood thinners this should not happen again. (Just one more thing to deal with)

Since I was the support person, I also had to learn how to give shots to Neil and what to look for in determining if there is a clot. I passed on actually giving him a shot and let Mary do it. Mary and I both learned a great deal, but with Neil as the patient, these were things we'd rather not have learned because it was at Neil's expense. He was so patient with us.

I remember when Mary and I thought he should drink more water to flush out his system. We kept encouraging him to drink more and more, and he kept saying it was too much. When he had his blood tests, it showed his electrolytes were way out of whack. His doctor said it was from too much water. Neil looked at us and said, "See, I told you two it was too much water, but you're always too busy playing nurse." That was the closest he ever got to complaining and after that, we tried not to over do anything.

Neil mentioned that he had back pain. I was immediately afraid as I'm sure he and Mary were too. Seems like something new was always coming up.

Updates continued: Neil started the new chemotherapy on Tuesday. It's a drug that has been released from research and is now on the market. This one will free him up somewhat, in that Mary won't have to record everything he does. Also, this chemo is in pill form, which he takes four in the morning and four at dinner. He still has to have a blood draw once a week, but if he travels he can arrange to have that anywhere. His reaction to the new drug has not been severe; mild nausea so far. His back pain is a constant issue. He would feel so much better if not for that. Please continue to pray for healing. This is a terminal cancer and we need a miracle. Neil also becomes discouraged. It seems if he takes one step forward he gets knocked back two. If it's not the cancer, it's the back pain, or the blood clots or the side effects, or personal issues; and soon *he'll have to have the liver stints replaced. He needs a touch of encouragement from God and prayer is so powerful, and that <u>makes all of you so important to his recovery.</u> Through your prayers, you are instruments of God by which He'll bring His healing touch. What an honor. James 5:13:16 says, "Is any one of you sick? He should call the elders of the church to pray over him and anoint him with oil in the name of the Lord. And the prayer offered in faith will make the sick person well; the Lord will raise him up. If he has sinned, he will be forgiven. Therefore confess your sins to each other and pray for each other so that you may be healed. The prayer of the righteous man is powerful and effective."*

Please remember to pray for my brother and for Mary, (affectionately referred to as nurse Ratchet) As hard as this is for Neil, it is equally as hard for Mary who is the other half of him. Thank you for your faithfulness in praying. Gaynel

Journal: His new chemo is in pill form with blood tests once a week. If only he felt good, he could travel or do something normal and fun. They've lost the wonderful life they had, but through it all you can see how they love each other and the faith they have in the Lord; whatever happens!

Neil's new chemo doesn't cause much in the way of side effects except mild nausea, but he is in pain. It's his back; I'm so sorry for his pain! When will this stop? I want him well again.

Neil fights depression, and it's no wonder, when we always seem to get bad news. I'm so scared. I pray constantly. Please help my brother, don't let him die. I love him so.

When Neil started this second chemo, we were on another high. Things became easier, since there were no journals where Mary had to document everything and no more weekly trips to chemo which took all day. They still had to go in for blood tests, but that was so much easier.

Neil Update Dec. 12, 2000: Thought I'd send an update before the holidays. Neil is doing very well on this new treatment. Side effects are very minimal. Even the back pain is less. So physically he is feeling fairly good. Of course with the holidays there is the melancholy that is somewhat normal, but imagine if you had cancer; and some of you do know. He tries to stay on top of it and Mary reminds him that every day is a "happy day". It is so wonderful to see how they work together on everything.

Although we won't know what effect this treatment is having on the tumor shrinkage until January when he has his next cat scan, his blood tests every week are looking very good. Please do not forget to pray for him and Mary. I'm a firm believer in the power of prayer and we need a miracle however the Lord chooses to bring it about. May God bless each of you and your families with health and happiness now and (I was going to say 'through the new year') forever! Happy holidays. PS: Believe in Miracles and the Power of Prayer! Gaynel

I continue to pray for Neil's healing and I do it with such passion; pleading, crying, interceding for him. When I kneel before the Lord in prayer, I actually feel like my heart is breaking. I want and expect Neil to be healed.

I'm always looking for something new, and I heard of how some research was being done with arsenic. I didn't know anything about it, so when we were at one of Neil's doctor appointments, I asked Dr. J about it and if it was something that could help Neil. He shook his head and made a sound or snicker that made me feel ridiculous, then he turned to Neil and said, "Well how about that Neil, would you like to put some arsenic in your body?" My big brother looked at him in all seriousness and said, "It can't be any worse than what you're putting in it." My hero. His comment lifted me right back up and put doc in his place. As I look back, I believe this was a turning place with Dr. J. Before this, he had welcomed all our questions and suggestions and openly talked with us about anything and everything. When Neil stopped responding to the chemo and it was obvious to the doctors that the end was near, we saw less and less of Dr. J. When we'd schedule appointments, he was often gone, or too busy and another doctor would cover for him. I really resented this and I know Neil was very hurt and discouraged. But then I have to try to put myself in the doctor's position. I can't imagine being an oncologist and not becoming attached to some patients more than others, and then losing them. A profession of saving lives in a field where many die. It has to be extremely difficult. I wondered then, and still do now, if Dr. J. was distancing himself from Neil at the end in order to protect himself from burning out in his line of work. Cancer affects so many people in so many ways, it's a ripple effect that keeps circling around. It's horrible.

Journal: It's Christmas time. Will it be our last with Neil? We all think he'll be here one or two more years; maybe we'll have a cure by then.

I remember that last July when the sister of one of the morning news anchors on a major network, was diagnosed with pancreatic cancer. Surely they must have resources none of us have. Maybe they'll find something. I grab at every straw I can. I can't let him die. There must be something, somewhere, I just have to find it. Lord help me find something.

Every year Neil and Mary spend the first weekend of December in Seattle. It's a special time for them to see all the decorations and do their Christmas shopping. They insist on living life fully and as normally as possible. Neil didn't feel great, but they went and did as much as possible. We went in for the day, and wouldn't you know it, Neil had managed to get an upgrade in his hotel room. It was a room that had been used as a 'president's suite'; a very nice room and a wonderful view.

They had Christmas, as always, with their four children and their spouses and their ten grandchildren who ranged in age from teens to a baby. Neil loved his family so much and enjoyed spending time with them. He and Mary often took the little ones to the ocean with them. He would hold baby Spencer all the time, and make noises to make him smile, and he'd play and read with the little girls, and the teens always looking forward to his great hugs.

Neil Update Dec. 28, 2000: Neil continues with his chemo. He had a one week break and is back at it now. The pill form is much easier to tolerate. The doctors told him to watch for soreness on the bottoms of his feet and fingertips. If he develops sores or cracking and/or blackness, they will take him off the chemo. He is noticing sensitivity there and is worried about problems developing, so he's using creams and lotions to keep his feet in good health. <u>He can't risk being taken off the chemo.</u> **Please pray about this.** *His blood tests, white and red counts and his tumor marker, continue to look good. His liver test is also good which means the stints aren't blocking up. For me it's hard to know what is going on without a cat scan, which we get Jan. 16.* **Pray for great results!**

Do you remember the saying that "a squeaky wheel gets the oil?" I feel like that. Not only with you, but with the Lord. I'm a nag (a squeaky wheel) and I don't apologize. I do and will continue to remind and plead with you to remember my brother in your prayers. He is so very dear to me and to all of us that love him so. As we were sitting in church Sunday, our pastor (he's great by the way, always seems to have a message just for me, probably because I need them!) anyway, our pastor was teaching and as usual I was thinking of Neil and praying for healing as I listened. Of course, we all know how God must have suffered because of the sacrifice of His son. Even as a babe in His mother's arms, God knew what lay ahead. Even watching Him as a young boy running and playing, God knew what lay ahead. And then enduring, while it happened to His only Son, knowing He could stop it only at the cost of our salvation. Wow! John 3:16 says,"For God so loved the world, that He gave His only begotten son, that whoever believes in Him should not perish, but have eternal life".

*Sometimes I think God doesn't know how bad this is for Neil and all of us. But as I sat there, I was hit with the reality of what God went through and what Jesus went through. Even feeling a small part of it, I was agonizing just as I agonize over Neil. I was aware that God personally knows my (our) anxiety, fear, pain, anger, hope, love…all the emotions involved. Not only because He endured it Himself, but I knew, I just knew that He personally feels what I'm experiencing. I was overwhelmed with the reality of it. You know how sometimes something that you've probably known forever just seems to sink in and become real. It gave me such a peace, knowing He knew what we were going through. I mean really knowing He knew. We're not alone in this. Even though we don't know what the outcome will be, all of us have our part to do in Neil's recovery. **Please continue to pray for healing.** It will be a miracle, God's glory. What a privilege for you to be a part of that! I appreciate all of you so much, your faithfulness to pray. May God bless us all with health and happiness in 2001. Embrace your family. Gaynel (The Squeaky Wheel)*

As they did every year, Neil and Mary went to the beach house for New Years. Neil's feet were bothering him very much by this time, but they still went out to dinner with their friends, and Neil even managed to give Mary a New Year's dance. He gave her one more wonderful memory.

We were all looking forward to the New Year 2001 with great and wonderful things happening in Neil's treatment and healing.

14

Side Effects of Chemo; Prayer for Help & God's Word

The hope of the new year did not last long; once again we were dropped down to the bottom of this roller coaster. It had been nine and a half months since Neil's diagnosis, and that entire time our emotions have taken every twist and turn possible, from the highest of highs to the lowest of lows. It's all very exhausting.

Neil Update Jan. 17, 2001: I just got home from going with Neil and Mary to his cat scan appointment yesterday. The news was not good. The tumors in Neil's liver are starting to come back. He will no longer be taking the chemo he was on since it is ineffective. He would have had to take a break from it anyway, because it has caused a great deal of damage to his feet and fingers. (a side effect) He is so very tired of never getting good news. Let me see if I can find a silver lining to this dark cloud. When Neil was taken out of the research program, his doctor told him there were two more drugs to try. One he preferred and another. We had to accept whatever the computer chose for him, and it was the other. NOW, we can have the treatment which the doctor preferred. It's called 'rubitecan'. Evidently it's derived from an herb and made into a drug. Mary found on the internet that some researchers are combining it with 'gemcitabine' (which was one of the drugs from the first research program that worked so well), and it's been effective on pancreatic cancer! So if it isn't effective by itself, we can ask to use the combination. This gives us yet another option. We hope to never run out of options!

Please be faithful in remembering to pray for my brother. He needs you so much. He and Mary love and trust in the Lord in all things, even this. But even so, they become discouraged and afraid. They need God's touch and protection. And a miracle!! I will never stop praying for that miracle healing. God bless you and your families. Thank you, thank you, thank you.

I don't think we ever understood why a computer got to pick which chemo Neil received first. I think it was all part of the research program he was in, and when one chemo failed they'd try the next, and there were only three. He was having such a hard time. His feet had turned black and the skin was peeling off, so of course it hurt to walk. His hands were also very sore. I can't tell you how much I hurt for him. And poor Mary, she was dying inside with anguish and fear. How do you stop this attack on someone you love? We pray and pray, and Neil is not getting better.

Neil Update Jan.23, 2001: Neil had another doctor appointment yesterday. Jed and I spent the weekend with them at the ocean. It was great just to be there with them. Neil was very tired and slept a lot and Mary had to cut a lot of black, dead skin off his feet. They were so badly burned from this last chemo, but they are healing up nicely now. Isn't it odd what we put into our bodies to kill the cancer......actually it kills everything, good and bad. Oh, the fight for life. God gave us the will to live, and a strong one it is! I asked the doctor about a new test drug used for leukemia that has arsenic in it. We can't help grabbling at straws.

Dr. J prescribed mega doses of vitamin B-6 to help heal his feet. He wants them well before he starts the 'rubitecan' next week. I say it's about time we put something in his body that will replenish and build up his own natural fighting resources.

Dr. J said that this is the last treatment they have for Neil. If it fails, we must look elsewhere for further options. **Let's pray this will put him into the remission we hope for.**

When we began this, we started looking for options that we could try if we reached this stage. I've read some wonderful stories about metabolic/nutritional/naturopathic treatments. Mary and Neil are going to look into working in this area now with someone that will work with his doctor. It only makes sense to give the body what it needs to help fight off this invasion of disease. **Please pray for God's touch of comfort, peace and healing for Neil, and to lead us in the right direction for treatment.**

We had such powerful prayer for Neil this weekend. God said he would send His Comforter, and we would be able to lay hands on the sick in Jesus name, and they would be healed. (look up 'healing' in your bible...you can read for hours) He said it, so it's true, right? Yes it's true. We actually prayed Neil to sleep, and asked for a healing sleep, and that he would wake up healed. I truly expected it. While he was sleeping, I asked Mary if she thought he would wake up healed. She said she didn't know, but she did know that He could heal Neil in the blink of an eye, that it could happen. We know this, our faith is strong, but we also know that good people die of cancer. Innocent children, young, old, believers and non. Why miracles for some and not oth-

ers? You pray with such faith and hope and nothing _seems_ to happen. Is it a test of faith? Could be…Job was certainly tested. The fact is, there are so many questions we have that we won't have answers for until we're in His presence. We must hold steadfast to our faith and not become discouraged. God doesn't make mistakes. I don't have the answers, but I know I love Him and trust Him, even and especially, in this. He'll see us through. **Keep praying for that miracle.**

Journal: We went to the ocean with Neil and Mary. Mary's afraid to go alone, in case Neil gets really sick and needs help. I feel so bad I can't help him. Mary and I prayed over him for an hour or more even after he fell asleep. I really expected him to wake up healed. Why God? I claim all Your promises of healing and faith and why aren't my prayers answered with healing?

Journal Jan. 28, 01 Sunday: Last night when I was praying for Neil, the Lord gave me a vision of him being raised up with the angels to heaven. It was so beautiful; but I cried and cried. This was the second time God told me Neil would go home. I pray with such agony and desperation that I believe God wanted me to rest and know that He has Neil in His care and will take him home. I slept very well that night, but when I woke I didn't want to accept it.
Today, in church, I was praying for Neil's healing (instead of listening) and that small, still voice of the Holy Spirit said in my head, "I'm bringing Neil home." This was the third time God told me!

I was exhausted. God wanted me to let go and rest, knowing that He held Neil in His loving care and it wasn't for me to decide, but I just couldn't let go. The Lord has told me three times, but I won't accept it. This is an example of that classic statement, "Let go and let God." Whose hands are we and our loved ones in, ours or God's? I'm so stubborn and He has such gentle patience with me!

Journal: I tried to accept it for about a day and then I realized that I could pray for God to change His mind! So my prayers have changed to that. My selfish prayer is, "don't take him home, heal him".

It's selfish because we all want him here, when in reality our greatest reward is to be in heaven. Neil deserves heaven after all this suffering. Not that any of us "deserve' heaven, we don't;' but for the grace of God through His son Jesus' we can have heaven. Even so, I still want Neil here for many years to come. Please change Your mind, heal him.

I can't tell anyone about Neil going home. Except Jed, I share everything with him. I don't want anyone to stop praying for healing. I hope it's not wrong for me not to tell, but that would be so hard for me. I pray that God will tell whoever needs to hear it.

Neil Update Sunday Jan. 28, 2001: Wanted to let everyone know that Neil is having a procedure on Tuesday to block the pain. His pain has increased in his side and back, so it is time for another pain block. They put a needle in his spine and shoot in alcohol to deaden the nerves. They've done this once before, but it is only temporary. Please pray that this will be very effective and that with less pain he can concentrate on his recovery. We are looking forward to the new treatment he will start this week, and hopeful that it will be successful. We thank you all for your prayers, (you can't possibly know how much they mean to Neil and Mary and how much they help). We sang a song in church today with words something like this: (I can't remember the exact words) 'I have a Father in heaven, He knows my name, He knows my thoughts, He feels my pain, He sees my every tear, He hears my every need.'
I'm overwhelmed whenever we sing it. It's so true that our God is all knowing, omniscient. He does hear your prayers, because you matter to Him. Thank you all for sticking with us through this. To Him be the glory.

Neil Update Feb. 2, 2001: Gaynel has asked me to send this Neil update, as she is at the hospital with Neil and Mary for probably the next three days. They had gone in this morning for the results of an MRI and to get a spinal pain block. At prayer this morning we believed there was going to be good news. But that proved to be not the case. The MRI showed a tumor on Neil's spine, and this is what was causing him so much pain in his back and legs. One option was for radiation on the cancer tumor, but that would delay or completely cancel his new chemo that he was to begin taking today. So, they are opting for the chemo which will work against all the tumors, wherever they are; pancreas, liver and the spine! This afternoon, Neil received a pain control devise that he can control and administer himself. Apparently it requires two or three days in the hospital to learn how to control it. This is why they are staying in. We have been praying for a miracle, and so far our Heavenly Father has not said yes, but He has not said no either. (He did to me, but I can't or won't tell anyone.) So please continue to intercede on Neil's behalf right into the Throne Room of the Lord of all Creation, Our Redeemer and healer, Jesus Christ! Every prayer helps. If the doctors can't do it, our Lord certainly can. A call of prayer and encouragement to Neil would, I am sure, be a blessing to him. We are so thankful for each and every one of you… THE LORD'S RICHEST BLESSING ON EACH ONE OF YOU. Hadley.

That day we went into the hospital for a doctor's appointment and the relatively simple pain block, knowing it would take most of the day, but planning on being home that afternoon. We were there for five days!

Mary and I had to learn how to operate the pain monitor, checking and cleaning it to make sure it isn't clogged, changing it when it empties and knowing what to do if it malfunctions. We have to watch for fevers, check for evidence of blood clots and simply be on top of anything and everything that may be going on. We've learned so much through this and none of it by choice.

Journal: Neil was supposed to get another spinal pain block but an MRI showed a tumor on his spine. Oh God please, I don't know what to do!

He was in so much pain. It was suddenly so much worse. He was laying there waiting for them to prepare to do a different kind of block. He hurt so bad he didn't know if he should lay or sit. I couldn't stand his pain and I fell apart. I went in the next room, obviously I was a mess, and I told them with a strong yet shaky voice, to hurry and do something because my brother is hurting. And to do it now!

I had to be strong in front of Neil, but when they took him into the procedure room, which they did right away, I dropped to the floor and fell apart. Mary was a mess too. This was the most pain we've ever seen Neil in; or the most he'd ever revealed to us. It was too much for us to handle. All through this we have been each other's support, and now we had to help each other and encouraged each other, knowing that we had to be strong and hold together for Neil's sake. And we did.

The procedure is a pump that puts morphine right on his spine.

Neil's pain is gone.

The day after Neil's procedure, he was feeling so good. He said he didn't have any pain and you could actually see the relief on his face.

Neil Update Feb 9, 2001: To the prayer warriors for Neil and Mary. It has been a most difficult time for Neil and Mary. About five days were spent in the hospital, and Neil was released on Monday afternoon the 5th, at about 4:30. The following morning he was back in because of shallow breathing. He spent the day in ER and later he was admitted as a patient. They discovered liquid in his lungs. They had earlier discovered blood clots in his legs and had thinned out his blood to help them dissolve, so they could not remove the liquid in his lungs until the blood was back to normal. On Thursday they were able to remove the liquid on one side and will do the other hope-

fully today. They don't think the infection in his body is serious, but they are giving him antibiotics.

All of this has been very difficult to handle for all of us, as it came on so fast, and we have been hoping and praying so hard for a miracle healing!

Sunday afternoon. It is now two days later. Neil did not have to have liquid removed from the other side of his lung. The doctor said there was not enough there to warrant any risk from extracting it. He is breathing better and resting, even with all the company! On Saturday, a hospital bed was set up for him in their home, and hospice care will be included to help Mary and give exercises to Neil to bring back strength to his legs and the rest of his body. He should be released from the hospital today or Monday. The doctor told Mary it would probably be down hill from this time on, but the Lord of miracles is still on call, and we are the one's He is expecting to hear from. It takes prayer; it takes prayer; it takes prayer.

Please be diligent during your times of prayer to remember Neil and Mary. The doctors may give up, because they are of limited knowledge and ability, but God is not. Maybe this is just the point of time when Our Lord Jesus Christ is ready. Keep going before His Throne petitioning for Neil's healing. Hadley

"May mercy and peace and love be multiplied to you." Jude 2

Jed came into the hospital on Sunday, Feb. 11th to be with us and help us get Neil home. It was almost Valentine's Day and Neil asked if we could get him something to give Mary. Oh, that just broke my heart. He loved her so much and was always thinking of her and others. Since we had to go pick up some medical items for Neil to have at home, we looked around for something. I spotted this little crystal angel holding a red heart in his hands. I picked it up and started crying. Neil gave that to Mary for Valentine's Day, along with the flowers that Neil arranged to have Kenny order for him.

15

The Final Days: Lord Help Me, I Can't Let Go

Neil Update Feb 12, 2001: My brother Hadley, bless his heart, has sent a couple of updates for you since I've been away from home. Jed and I just came home over night to get our motor home so we can stay with Neil and Mary. We did have hospice lined up to come in and help, but they will not assist if the patient is still receiving treatment. The doctors felt they would, since it is a 'compassion' treatment with a test drug at no cost to them, but they refused. We chose chemo over hospice. We're not quitters. They'll be available should we run out of options.

As Hadley told you, two weeks ago Neil went in for a two-hour procedure to block the pain and stayed in the hospital for almost two weeks with the exception of one night at home. They put an epidural in his back that puts a morphine cocktail directly to the tumor that is causing the leg and back pain. He can give himself an extra shot of it should he need too. It's been one complication after another; blood clots in his leg, fluid in his lungs, (they took almost two liters out of his right lung!), stabilizing his blood clotting levels, stabilizing the epidural pain meds, swelling of his legs from fluid retention! The epidural itself causing problems with the strength in his legs. He can barely walk. It also causes leg tremors and the meds for that make him sleepy. We pray, and pray and pray. Sometimes, I don't know how to pray. I just have to cry out for help. I pray, "If You won't heal him, won't You at least take away all the bad side effects and complications so the meds can do their best?" I wonder in God's infinite wisdom and mercy what I'm missing here. What is going on? Where are You?

Our faith is not at stake here. We don't have to understand to believe. God says to keep asking and petitioning, even if we don't receive. Keep praying, and we do. We know there is no cure for this cancer, but we hoped Neil would rally for a while on this new chemo. And he still might. Mary said he had a wonderful night last night and feels better this morning. (We grab at every glimmer of hope) God will see us through. We belong to Him and He holds us dear. Your prayers are vital, not only for that healing we want, but for protection, comfort, and understanding of all this that is beyond our ability. The Holy Spirit will show you how and what to pray. There are some of you, I know, who actually get woken up at night to pray for Neil, and many who the Holy Spirit taps on the shoulder during the day. See, God is with us, seeking prayers from you prayers. Thank you for your perseverance. We need your prayers.

I don't know if I can even explain what I'm going through during this time. I'm in a fog. Jed and I have our motor home in front of Neil and Mary's. We have our walkie talkies in case Mary needs us in the night. When she gets up every morning, she puts a little angel on the window sill so we know she's up. I do what I can to help, but she insists she will care for Neil. I do other things to help like laundry, cooking, dishes, those sorts of things.

Neil is in their bedroom in a hospital bed beside their bed. It's next to a sliding glass door to the patio and though it's still winter, I bought some early spring flowers and planted them in a pot outside his window. His kids bought an outdoor fireplace for the patio and they light it for him every night.

I had to call my brother Keith, and tell him he'd better come up and see Neil now. I won't believe he's dying; he still looks so good to me. Just another bump in the road! Keith flew up the next day and stayed for a week, close to Neil, and Hadley came every day. We all prayed with him and read to him and just talked.

Neil Update Feb. 14, 2001: Neil had a doctor's appointment today for his weekly blood and urine tests. He has these to determine if he is able to continue with his chemo. We had to transport him by ambulance, since his legs are still too weak for him to walk, and we have to keep his legs elevated because of swelling. Early this morning Mary discovered his epidural was leaking, so we were afraid they would have to keep him in the hospital to replace it. Thankfully, they were able to fix it quite easily. However, there was blood in his urine and his blood tests showed his electrolytes were too low, potassium too high, and his blood clotting time was too low. (I think that's all!) Because of these problems, he can't have any chemo this week in order to clear these things up. Also, Mary has to give him shots twice a day for his blood thinner. Since I'm the back-up support, I had to learn to give him his shot today. I acted like it was no big deal, but I have to tell you, it was so hard to poke my brother with that needle. He hurts enough as it is. (Maybe I should have pretended we were kids again!) He said I did a great job, and he didn't even feel it. This man is so wonderful. With all he's been through this last year, he always, and I mean always, thinks of everyone else and worries about how they're handling his cancer. He never complains and is so good natured about Mary and me fussing at him to do this and not that. It just breaks my heart that such a bad thing happened to such a nice man.

Please pray that: 1. next week when he has his blood test that everything will be OK for him to have his chemo. 2. that he will adjust to the epidural and regain strength in his legs. 3. that his new chemo will work for him in shrinking the tumors. 4. that he will not get more fluid in his lungs or blood clots. 5. that he will have no more bad side effects or complications. 6. that he will continue to feel the presence of our Lord's peace and comfort. 7. that the Holy Spirit will continue to bring Neil to people's minds for prayer. 8. for the miracle healing!

You know, sometimes we think our prayers are not being answered because Neil continues to get worse, but think about how God has touched so many through this. How Neil has maintained his courage, dignity, faith and gentle spirit through all of this. How Mary has been so brave and wonderful, rising to each new challenge successfully. It is only through the grace of God that we are able to endure. Your prayers have helped so much and will continue to help. Keep petitioning the Lord in Neil's behalf…He hears and He responds in His perfect way.

I'll probably never understand why things are the way they are, but I'll always believe in miracles!! Keep praying for them. God bless you and thank you so much.

I can't believe how much company is coming and going. There's almost a constant flow of people. They're all so sad. I know they think they are seeing Neil for the last time and it makes me mad because I refuse to think of him dying. He still looks so good to me! There's that anger again; it crops up at times when it shouldn't. I can't seem to turn it loose; and I can't accept heaven as the ultimate healing that I know it is. I know he's dying, even if I pretend he's not and I have no right to be angry at others for accepting it. I just don't want to see it. I keep trying to control this, keeping Neil in my hands, when all along he's been in God's hands. I have to let go of my fear and rely on my faith, because I'm also in God's hands.

Neil Update February 20, 2001: I'm using my daughter's computer again since we are still staying with Neil and Mary. Neil is still home and in a hospital bed. He gets up sometimes once a day and sits in his wheel chair. Yesterday his daughter Tammy came over and lovingly cut his hair. He sat up for quite a while before he was ready to go lay back down. Tomorrow he has a doctor's appointment, and we asked for a CT to see if they could withdraw some of the fluid in his abdomen. He is so bloated that it is difficult for him to move about. Once again, he will travel by ambulance.

He still has blood in his urine, so we know they will not give him his chemo again this week. We've been praying for a plan B for just this situation since last March, because we knew modern medicine offered no cure. We're in our final hours now and grabbing at straws. Our son Jason's wife, Jenny, heard of an unconventional treatment some people in our area were using, so Saturday I called to order some. It would take five days to get it because of the holiday. We talked about driving or flying to Idaho to get it, but my brother Keith felt the Lord tell him, "be still ye of little faith." Oh Lord, how you want us to trust You! We went to church Sunday and one of the things the pastor said was that we often <u>focus on our fear instead of our faith</u>! OK, that was me. Neil seemed to be weakening daily and I was so afraid that five days was too long to wait. Since Neil and Mary had our cousins staying with them, Jed and I drove home, to spend the night, and check on things there. All the way home, I prayed about this treatment, and asked the Lord if it was what we should do or not and if it was, to open the doors to it. I personally did not know anyone who had it, but Jenny had found some names and numbers, and the first phone call I made I got some. More than I needed until our order arrived. We drove straight back to North Bend.

Neil cannot have his chemo, but at least we are trying something. Doing nothing physically constructive is more than we can handle. We are constantly praying and <u>that is everything.</u>

How many times have I thought of sayings like,' pray and you shall receive'; 'if you do not receive it is because you have not asked'; 'petition to the Lord in His name';' pray with passion'; 'be specific in your prayers';' pray a certain way'; are my short comings standing in the way of God answering my prayers for Neil's healing?, on and on. We can all drive ourselves crazy with these things; doubts from the evil one, that's what these are.

God hears our prayers, all of them from all of us. Do not grow tired of praying and petitioning for Neil. Now it is most important and vital. Now is when a miracle will be fully recognized as truly that. God holds Neil firmly in His loving care. He knows our fears and pleas, He hears our petitions, He is always there for us, even when we cannot rest in Him and be calm, even when we focus on our fears and not our faith. Dear Lord, help me to do that. Help me to place Neil totally in Your hands. Let me rest in You and focus on You as I continue to stand in the gap for Neil and petition, plead and pray for Your healing touch that will restore Neil to the perfect health You created in him.

Please pray like crazy now. Our God is an awesome God. Let's watch Him continue to work in this. Thank you all and God Bless you. Do you realize you've become prayer warriors? Gaynel

I wonder now, as I look back, just how crazy it was to try something that we'd heard about, but knew nothing about, except that it worked for one person we knew of. We were desperate and we all talked it over, including Neil and we decided it wouldn't hurt anything now because Neil was dying, regardless. It was a paste of herbs very, very condensed and concentrated. Keith and I both tried some before we gave Neil any. It was all we had left to try.

Keith went to Neil's last doctor's appointment with us, then left for the airport from the hospital. Neil, once again, was transported by ambulance.
The doctor told Neil it was too hard for him to go back and forth and that he didn't need to continue with his appointments. He was giving up on him.

Journal: Neil's off chemo and hospice in involved. They're wonderful.
Keith was here for a few days. The day he flew home he went to the hospital with us. (Neil's last visit) Dr. J was not there again and we saw a doctor we had not seen before. He asked Neil what they could do for him, meaning to make him comfortable, and Neil said, "Give me ten more years and I'll coast from there"! Neil never gave up!

Of course the doctor thought we were all in denial and was very concerned about us. We assured him that we knew the gravity of the situation and that Neil was dying, but that we were Christians and we always had hope.

Journal: Keith liked to sit and read to Neil even when he was sleeping. I often did this too, just so he knew we were there.
Mary takes such good care of him. She won't let nurses or anyone else care for him. She does it all!
Neil became <u>very</u> bloated in his abdomen. He was huge. An effect of the cancer certainly, but was it one of the signs in the final stage? Was his body shutting down? I was so afraid.

At Neil's doctor appointment, they did drain his abdomen, and that made a huge difference in his comfort level. He had gotten so bloated around the middle that Mary had to buy him new pants. She found that the 'break away' pants, with snaps down both sides, were the easiest to get on and off of him. Neil couldn't get up anymore and needed total care. He was still alert, though he tired easily and he was still eating and drinking.

I remember the morning after Neil first took the paste. He had a catheter in and had a urine bag, and that morning for the first time there was no blood in his urine. I was so happy, I just knew it was from the new 'paste'. It was such a good sign. Mary was excited too, but she reminded me that it could have been because they had drained the fluid off his abdomen the previous day and the pressure had let up on his organs. I wanted to believe it was because this 'paste' was reversing all the effects of the cancer and he was getting better.

The day before at the hospital they told us that Neil would not be getting anymore chemo and they advised us to call hospice. We agreed and they helped us get them set up to come out. We weren't telling anyone about the 'paste' that I thought was going to make him better. Wouldn't they be surprised?!

The nurse took me aside in the hall and told me she was concerned that we weren't prepared for what was going to happen. She told me that Neil's time was very short. A matter of days and he would probably go into a coma; and she told me different things to look for. She also said that Mary and I would probably get ill because our stress had more than likely knocked out our immune system. She said she saw that often happen to the care givers and close family members. Mary and I immediately took measures to fortify ourselves; we didn't want to risk getting sick and passing it onto Neil.

Journal: I still think Neil is going to get better. He has too! This isn't real. It can't be happening!

February 25th was not unlike any of the others days that had fallen into our pattern, with the regular chores, company and spending quality time with Neil. He slept a lot, but was alert and visited with us during the day and during his meals. After we had dinner that night with Neil and Mary, we stayed and waited while Mary cared for Neil's needs, helping him get ready for bed. We always stayed in the evenings in case she needed us for anything. We retired to our motor home about 9:00 p.m. and went straight to bed. It didn't take long for the walkie talkie to start making noises. We discovered that sometimes other people would come within range of our signal and we would pick them up. The walkie talkie kept going off, but no one ever came on the line. I finally got suspicious and scared at the same time. When it went off again, I pushed the button and asked if it was Mary. She said, "Yes, please hurry I need help with Neil". She thought by signaling us on the walkie talkie we would come right in, but because she didn't talk, we thought it was someone else.

Journal: Feb. 25 Mary called us into the house after we had gone to the motor home for the night. Neil was thrashing about and we couldn't get through to him or calm him.

Neil was completely out of it. We couldn't hold him down and he wouldn't respond to us. He had just talked with us, and said good night; he said he'd see us in the morning. Although he had been declining, it seems like this just happened too fast.

Journal: We called hospice and the nurse came quickly. She called the doctor on call and asked the service to have him call her immediately. She only waited a short time, with Neil in such distress, before she started forcing as many pills down him as she could. I thought she was going to kill him with an overdose! Can you imagine, I still wouldn't accept that he was dying!
Neil calmed down and settled. The doctor called and confirmed that she did the right thing to calm Neil so he could rest peacefully. She left after telling us that if he started to thrash about again to force his pills down him.

After the nurse left, Jed and Mary and I prayed by Neil's bedside and stayed with him for a while almost in shock. We had just had dinner with him and said good-night, see you in the morning. What in the world had happened? I knew this was happening, but it was like I wasn't really there. I was in a fog and it was too thick to come out of. Jed and I both cried back in the motor home and we both had to face up to the fact that this was the end.

Journal: The next morning Neil started thrashing about again and Mary and I had to force pills down him. How hard this was for both of us. God, where are You? Help us! Neil settled down again and remained calm.

As the day progressed, we knew we had to call everyone back. I remember how heavy it all was; the air, the atmosphere, everything was just so heavy and pressing down on me. I felt like I was moving in slow motion. I wanted to be with Neil the whole time, but there were just too many people who also wanted to be with him. I had to step aside and allow time for everyone else.

And so the day became evening with no change in Neil. He was peaceful and in a coma. We all talked to him, and Kerry, his son, played a song for him that he had written. This was the last goodbye.

We knew this was the end. Neil's son Jerry had just left Sunday and was now driving back. We prayed he'd make it before Neil died. Brian (our nephew) *was up north somewhere and was hurrying too, as soon as he heard. The house was full; Jed and I, Lia and Gary* (our daughter and one of our sons. Our other son, Jason wasn't able to be there) *Hadley and his family, all of Neil's kids and grandkids and his mother-in-law, Millie. I'm not sure who else, it's a blur to me. The hospice nurse was there for a while, but left after giving us instructions of what to expect and to call her when we needed to.*

I remember her talking with Hadley. He said, "It's so hard because this is all out of order. I'm supposed to go first." I guess the oldest expects that, but life isn't that orderly, nor is death. There are no rules for death; and no control over it.

We were always by his bedside; in and out throughout the day and night, each spending special moments with him. Kerry played a tape of one of his songs. I know Neil was very proud of him. He was very proud of all his kids. We all talked with him and around him. He knew we were there and he didn't go home until everyone was there. I wanted so badly to stop it and see that miracle I'd always prayed for, but it didn't happen.

What did happen for me was before he died, when I felt such a strong presence of the Holy Spirit. All I could do was stand by Neil's bed and praise God. Can you imagine, my brother was dying and I was praising God. I could have been angry with Him for not healing Neil, but instead I was praising Him. This in itself was an answer to prayer. Not the answer I wanted, but one just the same. Praising God is such a wonderful healing balm for us when we are hurting and don't understand. It puts us in His presence where all is well. A respite.

Neil had continued to remain calm and the only change that occurred was near the end when his breathing became very shallow and raspy. He died peacefully at 11:25 p.m. on February 26, 2001. He was only 55 years old.

When he died, I stopped praising God. I sensed and actually knew that Neil and the angels had left. I felt it. They were all gone. The room was full of people and yet empty.

Journal: I wept and wept and wept, in Jed's arms, when he died. Then I was so drained I sat on the floor and cried a bit more, but I was empty. After some time, I got up and took a few steps out of the room and collapsed into sobs. Jed and Gary knelt beside me and just let me fall apart.

I was unaware of whom or what was going on around me. I've always assumed the role of care giver, but for the first time I could only concentrate on my own loss; and it was overwhelming.

Journal: It doesn't matter how long you expect death, the finality of it is overwhelming. Being a Christian, I know death is not final. Yes, Neil's body died, but he did not. I'll see him again, <u>but even knowing this,</u> death is so hard. I can't imagine facing death without Christ and eternity in heaven. Neil's body died and he just moved to his heavenly home and I'll see him and mom and dad when I get there. It doesn't get any better than that! Eternity in paradise in the very presence of God Almighty. Wow! Many times after his death, when I was feeling my loss and so very sad, I would think of this, of where he was and imagine what it must be like for him and it made me feel so much better.

Neil Update: Neil passed away last night at 11:25 p.m.. It was peaceful and all the family was there with him. Thank you all for your prayers and support. Please keep my Aunt Mary and her family in your prayers as she has just lost her best friend, and they have lost the most wonderful father and grandfather. It's a comfort and joy to know where he is now, but it certainly doesn't ease all the pain we feel in losing him so soon. He was the most precious man! I'm feeling very dried up and emotionally spent right now. It's been a long day and night. God bless you all and thank you. Lia

Neil Update: I know that many of you already know of Neil's passing last night at 11:25, but I had to write one last update. One I hoped to never write. You were all so vital to Neil's battle. Please don't ever under estimate the power of your prayers. Our prayers weren't answered the way we wanted, but they were answered in so many other ways. Neil had 11 months to prepare himself and all of us for this time. And it was precious time. We took Neil to the hospital last Wed. and the doctor asked Neil what he expected at this point in his treatment. (The doctor was referring to pain management and what Neil expected at the end.) Neil told him, 'another ten years, then I'll coast from there'! The doctor wasn't ready for that answer. He thought we were all in total denial. But it was just like Neil to give him an honest answer! I can't imagine being in a world without hope, especially when the world offers no hope. Christians always have hope, even when our prayers aren't answered like we want. Neil was with us until the last 26 hours or so before he went into a coma. The hospice nurses were amazed at that. Because of your prayers, Neil was able to hold in there with us. He told us once that when the time came, he wanted to be in a big bed with all his grandkids piled around him. He didn't have a big bed, but his entire family, kids, grandkids, brother, sister, nieces, nephews, mother-in-law, and his precious wife were with him the whole time. His passing was very peaceful. He was surrounded by all the sounds that large families make; a sound that was certainly a comfort to him. Another answer to your prayers. I can't even begin to understand why this happened, but while I was standing around my brother's bed, I simply had to praise God Almighty. I couldn't pray any more, but needed to praise God. After Neil was gone, I was overwhelmed at knowing he was in the presence of God, seeing the face of Jesus and totally surrounded by the very essence of all that is holy. Wow. It still amazes me to think of it.

Our prayers were answered all along, in the ways God knew we needed them to be. Please pray for Mary now. She's never been totally alone before. From her childhood family to her own family, she's always had someone living with her. No one and nothing can totally comfort her now except 'The Comforter'. Please remember her in your prayers for a long time. Thank you all, you prayer warriors. Where would we have been without you? Gaynel

Do you think we all prayed in vain, without an answer to our prayers and pleading?

Journal: As I look back I realize and can see how God was answering our prayers all along. No, Neil wasn't cured or healed but God was with him and us every step of the way. He gave us all the strength we needed and so much, much more.

I've learned over time and from the deaths of loved ones, that when I grieve it's not for them, but rather for my own loss. How can I grieve for them when they are home eternal in heaven? No, my grief is for me, for the hole left in my life without them. Every time I lose someone, a little piece of me dies too. I'll be whole again when we're all united in paradise.

Ultimately, Neil was healed. He has a new, perfect, heavenly body that will never see disease, pain or death. He has reached the goal; life eternal in the presence of God that is a gift through His son Jesus Christ.

16

No More Pain; Home Is Heaven

Neil's funeral was the next Saturday. We spent the rest of the week making preparations and going through the motions of getting ready. Bob and Ann, our cousins from Reno flew up to help us get through this time and Keith came back to his hometown to bury his little brother. And we cried.

I'll always remember when we left the church to drive to the cemetery, the radio was on and Travis Tritt was singing, "It's A Great Day To Be Alive"! Can you imagine the irony in that? But as I listened to that song, I got a big smile on my face and just knew, that would have been exactly what Neil would have told all of us. He also would have said, as he did many times, "Get Over It!"

When we were at the cemetery, a local businessman came up to me to give his condolences. He said he almost felt guilty being there because he was winning his battle with prostate cancer. I told him that Neil had prayed for him and his recovery and healing of the cancer, and that he should never feel guilty for surviving. His surviving cancer didn't keep him from dying, it just postponed it and if Neil hadn't died now, he still would have at a different time. We will all stand before our Lord someday to give an accounting. Are you ready? Death is inevitable, even though we'd rather it was later than sooner, we just don't know.

If you're not ready and want to accept the gift of eternal life just repeat this prayer with a sincere heart.

Dear Father, I come to you in Jesus' Name. I'm sorry for my sins.
I want to be forgiven and cleansed and made pure.
Forgive me now. I believe Jesus is who He says He is—God' Son.
I believe He rose from the grave and is alive in heaven now.

I invite You into my heart as Lord of my life.

Thank you for saving me. Thank you for eternal life! Amen

Now go tell someone the good news! Romans 10:9 says, "…that if you confess with your mouth Jesus as Lord, and believe in your heart that God raised Him from the dead, you shall be saved."

For you, Neil will end with this book, but for those of us who knew him and loved him, he will forever be in our hearts.

At our father's funeral eight years before, we started what I suppose has now become a funeral tradition for us, since we did it at Mom's and now Neil's. The kids and grandkids each take time to reflect and write down one of their fond memories.

I'll end this journey by sharing these memories with you, so that you might have an inkling of this wonderful man that is my brother.

It is my prayer for you that something in this story has helped you come to grips with your own unbearable journey. Always remember, that you are not alone now, and you never have been. He's right there. Embrace the Lord, and receive all the good things He has for you. The sun will shine again, just take it one day at a time. As hard as it is, and even if you don't feel like it's true, remember Psalms 118:24, "This is the day which the Lord has made: Let us rejoice and be glad in it".

Remembrances Of Neil Rogers

Kerry (son): If I could be half the man my father was, I would be satisfied. Men like my father aren't in great quantities in this world. He was my father, my friend and my hero. He smashed the wall I had built around my heart as a little boy, and I learned to love and trust again. It didn't happen overnight, but he never stopped trying, and I didn't exactly make it easy for him at times. I try every day to be like my dad: caring, compassionate, friendly and cheerful. It's not always an easy thing to do when it doesn't come naturally to you like it did with my dad. Now I have to somehow try and fill this giant void in my life. I've lost my hero. Who's going to save me now? All I can do is remember that someday we'll be together again.

Patti (daughter-in-law): I will always cherish my times with Neil. He was a wonderful father-in-law. He was a man that I truly admired and respected. I will miss him greatly and I loved him with all my heart and soul. Thank you for being a part of my life. Thank you for showing my husband how wonderful a marriage can be. You are leaving a legacy of love and understanding, even though you are leaving us too soon.

Sean (grandson): I remember one time Grandpa and I were at the beach. We were lying in the sand together and Grandpa spotted a shooting star and it turned into a meteor shower. Just me and him. I love him very much and I'll miss him.

Matthew (grandson): I loved Papa and I loved spending time with him at the beach house.

Tammy (daughter): I was 8 years old when my mom married my dad. Soon afterward he adopted Kerry, Jerry and me. When I was 10, Kenny was born and when someone at my school called him my half brother it made me so angry and I said, "he's just my brother." After that time I didn't want to tell people that I was adopted because they made it seem like it was somehow less of a family. To me it is more special because my dad didn't have to adopt me, he **wanted** to. He always treated me the way I know he saw me, as his daughter. He would even kid about different traits or characteristics that I inherited from him. When I became a Christian it was easier for me to understand God's love and willingness to adopt me as one of His own because of what my dad had already done. He forever blessed my life by the kind of dad he was and by how wonderfully he treated my mom. "Long ago…God chose us to be his very own, through what Christ would do for us; His unchanging plan has always been to adopt us into his own family by sending Jesus Christ to die for us. And He did this because He wanted to!" Ephesians 1:4&5

Christina (granddaughter): Grandpa loved to tease us. I remember when he told us that we could go pick out a baby bunny at Auntie Gaynel's house and take it home. Of course our mom said no, so we ended up leaving crying. Grandpa liked to go looking for sand dollars at the beach even though they already had a ton of them. He really liked being at the beach. I will always think of him there.

Nichole (granddaughter): My favorite times with Grandpa were at Christmas. He would read the Christmas story to us and let us put ornaments on the tree and we got to be Santa and pass out the presents. I also liked playing horseshoes with him at the beach even though he would always beat me. I will miss him teasing me about my boyfriends and my clothes.

Blake (grandson): I liked going to the beach with Grandpa and Grandma. We went for walks on the beach and collected shells. We played out in the sand fort and got wet and muddy all the time.

Jerry (son): I couldn't possibly put a lifetime of fond memories into a single day. Dad loved to take the family camping. My favorite place was Fish Trap Lake in Spokane. Dad would take us kids out fishing, and he never got mad when we got our lines all tangled up, or dropped our poles in the lake. It seemed we always caught a lot of fish. He would even let us take the boat out by ourselves on occasion. One particular trip we caught so many fish that someone came up with the idea of passing out the fish late at night to the other campsites. They called themselves the 'fish fairies'.

Karen (daughter-in-law): My favorite memories of Neil are when he showed me how to clean clams and drink margaritas out of a bottomless glass, and getting up early to go tide pool hunting in rubber boots while still in my pajamas.

Casey (granddaughter): Grandpa and I went for a walk on the beach. About halfway into the walk we went to sit down on a big rock in the middle of the wet sand. I **know** I saw a snake go under that rock, but Grandpa told me, "there are no snakes at the beach." After we sat down, Grandpa stuck his walking stick in the ground and two snakes came out from under the rock. Grandpa jumped farther than I did and almost tripped over his walking stick. I tried to ask him what he said again about the snakes. All of a sudden, he couldn't remember!

Allison (granddaughter): At Wapato Point I was the only one that wanted to go out on the boat. Grandpa took me out on the lake and after a while we stopped. My favorite song, "Rock Around the Clock" was playing on the radio, and I went swimming with my life jacket on and a rope tied from my life jacket to the boat.

Kenny (son): My dad was such a great person; there is no word to describe him. He will forever be the 'king of upgrades'. He always had the best views (even in the hospital) and received the best service. I know it was because he never talked down to people, but instead talked with them. One of my favorite memories of dad was cooking with him on the line. He always watered down the chili and the stew and said "food cost, food cost." He was a good cook and teacher. All the waitresses seemed to work a little faster when he was on the line. He would say things like, "busy hands are happy hands, a clean ship is a happy ship, you can't sell any apples out of any empty apple barrel, and if you've got time to lean, you've got time to clean." People didn't stand around when he was working. Everywhere he went, people naturally wanted to please dad and he always let them know how much they were appreciated.

With mom, he was so good to her, and so lost without her. One time mom went on a prayer weekend so Teri and I took dad to church. When we went to kneel down, we noticed he still had on his slippers.

My dad will be forever in my heart. There will be no greater compliment that if someone says, "you remind me of your dad."

Teri (daughter-in-law): I have had the privilege of knowing and loving a generous and kind Neil. He set a great example as a father and husband. Kenny is just like his dad! Neil helped raise such a good son for me to love. I am so blessed to have such a wonderful life that he has influenced in so many ways. I am so thankful our children were able to know their Papa. Although they are still so little, they have so many wonderful memories to hold on to. One of my personal favorite memories was going to the beach on Memorial Weekend. Neil, Mary, Kenny, Travis, and Todd went over Thursday and us girlfriends (Teri, Tracy, and Mandy) showed up on Saturday. We listened to great music. I think we heard 'Diamonds on the Soles of Her Shoes' a hundred times. We played volleyball and shot pool. It was so much fun. It seems like yesterday, and whenever I hear that song, I think of the very special weekend. One of the neatest things is that all us kid-couples ended up married. I will miss Neil every day and I will especially miss his hugs. He never said hello to me with out a hug, or goodbye without a hug and an "I love you". I always felt so loved when I received them and if ever there was anything wrong, his hugs comforted me. How could there be such power in a hug? The answer is that they were so genuine…the best hugs ever.

Karli (granddaughter): My favorite times with Papa were when we would take walks together.

Jennifer (granddaughter): I always loved feeding the birds with Papa.

Spencer (grandson): Papa made the best noises that would make me smile. It always worked!.

Further Reading

As I mentioned in the book, *A Cancer Battle Plan,* By Anne Frahm and Dave Frahm, was of help to me in that it laid out an alternative course. I have no way of knowing what is right for you in your battle, but I had to look at everything I could find.

After my sister-in-law, Audrey, lost her battle with breast cancer, the family was given the book, *Heaven, My Father's House,* by Anne Graham Lotz, which was very helpful to all of us.

I cannot suggest strongly enough that you read scripture. It will be of great comfort. If you are not familiar with reading scripture don't be intimidated by it. We've all had to learn our way through the Bible, and it can be overwhelming! Before you read, ask God to open your heart to His word and to give you an understanding of His word. You might want to start with the gospels, which are Matthew, Mark, Luke and John in the new testament; and the Psalms have always been a great comfort to me.

I will list a very few scripture references that I found helpful through this very difficult time. If I listed them all, that would be overwhelming too! Also, in the back of your Bible you can look up words, such as healing, salvation, prayer, or whatever you want to read about, and it will direct you to scripture relating to that. God Bless you in your reading.

Job 1:22 and Job 5:8

Psalm 51, Psalm 31:14, Psalm 55:22, Psalm 35:15 and Psalm 35: 17-18

1 Peter 5:6-7

Philippians 4:6-7 and Philippians 4:13

Romans 8: 26-28

James 5: 14-16

0-595-34374-0